Focused Operations Management for Health Services Organizations

Boaz Ronen
Joseph S. Pliskin
with Shimeon Pass

Foreword by Donald M. Berwick

Focused Operations Management for Health Services Organizations

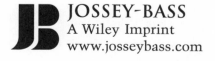

JOSSEY-BASS
A Wiley Imprint
www.josseybass.com

Published by Jossey-Bass
A Wiley Imprint
989 Market Street, San Francisco, CA 94103-1741   www.josseybass.com

Jossey-Bass books and products are available through most bookstores. To contact Jossey-Bass directly call our Customer Care Department within the U.S. at 800-956-7739, outside the U.S. at 317-572-3986, or fax 317-572-4002.

Jossey-Bass also publishes its books in a variety of electronic formats. Some content that appears in print may not be available in electronic books.

Library of Congress Cataloging-in-Publication Data

Ronen, Boaz.
  Focused operations management for health services organizations / Boaz Ronen, Joseph S. Pliskin, with Shimeon Pass ; foreword by Donald M. Berwick.— 1st ed.
      p. ; cm.
  Includes bibliographical references and index.
  ISBN-13: 978-0-7879-8454-0 (cloth : alk. paper)
  ISBN-10: 0-7879-8454-X (cloth : alk. paper)
  1. Health services administration.
  I. Pliskin, Joseph S., 1946-   II. Pass, Shimeon, 1947-   III. Title. [DNLM:
1. Health Services Administration.   W 84.1 R772f 2006]
  RA971.R566 2006
  362.1068—dc22   2006007386

Printed in the United States of America
FIRST EDITION
PB Printing   10 9 8 7 6 5 4 3 2 1

Contents

Figures and Tables   vii

Foreword   xv
Donald M. Berwick

Preface   xxi

About the Authors   xxv

Part One: The Dynamic Health Care Management Environment

1. The Modern Health Care and Business Environment   3

2. Principles of Management in a Dynamic Environment   11

3. The Pareto Rule, Focusing Table, and Focusing Matrix   29

Part Two: Novel Management Approaches

4. Management by Constraints: The Focusing Steps of the Theory of Constraints   47

5. Management by Constraints in a Bottleneck Environment   75

6. Management by Constraints When the Market
   Is the Constraint   99
7. Focused Current Reality Tree   119
8. Resolving Managerial Conflicts   131
9. The Efficiencies Syndrome   143
10. The Evils of Long Response Times   149
11. Reducing Response Times   163
12. The Complete Kit Concept   191
13. Performance Measures and Managerial Control   205
14. Effects of Fluctuations, Variability, and
    Uncertainty on the System   219
15. The Evils of Traditional Cost Accounting   237
16. Marketing, Costing, and Pricing Considerations
    in Decision-Making Processes   245
17. Quality Management and Process Control   263

Part Three: Strategy and Value Creation
18. Creating Value for Health Care Organizations   281

Part Four: Summary
19. Case Study: The Emergency Department at Guard
    Mountain Hospital   309
20. Our Managerial Credo   323

References   337
Index   341

Figures and Tables

Figures

Figure 1.1.   "Scissors Diagram" of Needs
              Versus Budget   8
Figure 1.2.   The Input-Output Model   9
Figure 2.1.   A Traditional Organizational
              System   12
Figure 2.2.   A Modern Organizational System   13
Figure 2.3.   The Satisficer's Approach   16
Figure 2.4.   Decision-Making Process: Optimizer
              Versus Satisficer   17
Figure 2.5.   Focused Management Triangle   20
Figure 2.6.   Classifying Problems by Their
              Contribution to the Organization   24
Figure 3.1.   Pareto Diagram   32
Figure 3.2.   Pareto Diagram of Analysis of
              Drug Costs   33
Figure 3.3.   Focusing Matrix for the ED Example
              in Table 3.3   39

Figure 4.1.   System Processes   52

Figure 4.2.   A System with a Resource
               Constraint   52

Figure 4.3.   A System with a Market Constraint   57

Figure 4.4.   A Process Flow Diagram   63

Figure 4.5.   A Two-Dimensional Process Flow
               Diagram   64

Figure 4.6.   A System and Its Work Process   67

Figure 4.7.   CUT Diagram of a System with
               a Resource Constraint   68

Figure 4.8.   CUT Diagram of a System with a
               Market Constraint   70

Figure 4.9.   CUT Diagram of a System
               with a Dummy Constraint   71

Figure 5.1.   Exploiting and Utilizing the
               Resource   76

Figure 5.2.   A Pareto Diagram of Specific
               Contribution   85

Figure 5.3.   The Drum-Buffer-Rope Mechanism   91

Figure 5.4.   Continuous Improvement in a Surgical
               Department   97

Figure 6.1.   Exploiting a Market Constraint   102

Figure 7.1.   Template for a Focused Current
               Reality Tree   120

Figure 7.2.   Cause-Effect Relation Between
               Undesirable Effects   123

Figure 7.3.   Example of a Cause-Effect Relation
               Between Undesirable Effects   123

Figure 7.4.   An "Extensive *Or*" Logical Relation   123

Figure 7.5.   Example of an "Extensive *Or*" Logical
                Relation of Undesirable Effects   124

Figure 7.6.   A "Logical *And*" Relation of
                Undesirable Effects   124

Figure 7.7.   Example of a "Logical *And*" Relation   125

Figure 7.8.   A Logical Loop Relation   125

Figure 7.9.   Example of a Loop Relation Between
                Undesirable Effects   125

Figure 7.10.   Example of Inference   126

Figure 7.11.   Example of an fCRT   128

Figure 8.1.   Dealing with Conflicts   133

Figure 8.2.   A Conflict Resolution Diagram   134

Figure 8.3.   A CRD for Service Variety   135

Figure 8.4.   A CRD for the Car Fleet Example   136

Figure 8.5.   A CRD for the Software Development
                Example   137

Figure 8.6.   Example of an Injection in a CRD   138

Figure 8.7.   A Public Hospital Outpatient Clinic
                with the Conflict of Treating Maximally
                Versus Treating Satisfactorily   138

Figure 8.8.   A Private Hospital Operating Room
                (OR) Scheduling Conflict of Volume
                Versus Flexibility   139

Figure 8.9.   Conflict in an Emergency
                Department (1)   139

Figure 8.10.   Conflict in an Emergency
                Department (2)   140

Figure 8.11.   Conflict of Errors Versus Cost in an
Emergency Department   140

Figure 8.12.   Clinical Conflict in Diagnosis   140

Figure 8.13.   Conflict in an OR: What to Do
with Patients   141

Figure 8.14.   Flexibility Conflict in OR
Scheduling   141

Figure 9.1.   A 1-2-3 Process and Department
Utilization   144

Figure 10.1.   Types of Inventories   150

Figure 10.2.   A High-WIP Center (A) Versus a
Low-WIP Center (B)   151

Figure 10.3.   Effect of the Forecasting Horizon on
Forecasting Quality   157

Figure 10.4.   Effect of Reducing WIP on
Organization Function and Value   161

Figure 11.1.   A 1-2-3 Production System with
Three Products   170

Figure 11.2.   Violation of JIT Rule I   171

Figure 11.3.   Response Time of a 1-2-3 System
with a Transfer Batch of Twenty-
Five Units   174

Figure 11.4.   Response Time of a 1-2-3 System
with a Transfer Batch of Five Units   175

Figure 11.5.   Working with Large Working
Batches   177

Figure 11.6.   Working with Smaller Working
Batches   177

Figure 11.7.   Negative Effects of Bad Multitasking   184

Figure 11.8.   System Arrangement with Functional
Structure   186

Figure 11.9.   System Arrangement Using
Group Technology Approach   187

Figure 11.10.   The Claims Department Before
Group Technology   188

Figure 11.11.   The Claims Department After
Applying Group Technology   188

Figure 12.1.   Conflict Resolution Using a
Complete Kit   197

Figure 14.1.   The Planned Process   221

Figure 14.2.   A CUT Diagram for Alternative A   222

Figure 14.3.   A CUT Diagram for Alternative B   222

Figure 14.4.   A CUT Diagram for Alternative C   223

Figure 14.5.   Alternative A with Internal and
Cumulative Fluctuations   225

Figure 14.6.   Alternative B with Internal and
Cumulative Fluctuations   225

Figure 14.7.   Alternative C with Internal and
Cumulative Fluctuations   226

Figure 14.8.   A Separate Line for Every Product   233

Figure 14.9.   A Common Core for Several Products
(Mushroom Effect)   233

Figure 16.1.   A CUT Diagram for Blood Tests   251

Figure 16.2.   A Core Competence Matrix   253

Figure 16.3.   Demand Curve for the Service
Mix Example   258

Figure 17.1.   Adding Inspection at the End of
                the Line   269

Figure 17.2.   A Closed-Loop Control System   270

Figure 17.3.   The Ten-Times Rule   273

Figure 18.1.   A Focused Current Reality Tree
                for Queen Medical Center   299

Figure 18.2.   Focusing Matrix for Value
                Enhancement at Queen Medical
                Center, Based on Table 18.3   306

Figure 19.1.   The Traffic Light Zones   315

Figure 19.2.   Focused Current Reality Tree
                for the ED   318

Figure 19.3.   Focusing Matrix for the ED Action
                Items, Based on Table 19.1   319

Tables

Table 3.1.   Drug Use Volume and Costs in a
              Hospital Ward   32

Table 3.2.   Classification by Drug Costs   33

Table 3.3.   Emergency Department (ED)
              Focusing Table   39

Table 4.1.   Labor Hours per Unit per Station   65

Table 4.2.   Load Analysis   66

Table 4.3.   Load Analysis with a Bottleneck   68

Table 4.4.   Load Analysis in a System with a
              Market Constraint   69

Table 4.5.   Load Analysis in a System with
              a Dummy Constraint   71

Table 5.1.   Imaging Projects   84

Table 6.1.   The Specific Contribution of Customers
               Relative to the Sales Effort   105

Table 11.1.   Effect of Batch Size on the Load of
               Noncritical Resources   180

Table 13.1.   Calculation of Throughput   209

Table 13.2.   Due Date Performance Using the
               Dollar-Days Measure   213

Table 13.3.   The Measurements Profile   216

Table 15.1.   Loss of Relevance of the Assumptions
               Underlying Traditional Cost
               Accounting   243

Table 16.1.   Measurements Profile for a Make-or-
               Buy Decision   252

Table 16.2.   Measurements Profile for the
               Production Example   256

Table 16.3.   Demand as a Function of Price   257

Table 16.4.   Measurements Profile for the Service
               Mix Example   259

Table 18.1.   Return on Assets (ROA) and
               Economic Value Added (EVA)   286

Table 18.2.   Analysis of Queen Medical Center's
               Strengths, Weaknesses, Opportunities,
               and Threats   295

Table 18.3.   Focusing Table for Queen Medical
               Center Value Drivers   305

Table 19.1.   Focusing Table for the ED
               Action Items   319

Table 19.2.   Action Items for Teamwork   320

Foreword

Health care organizations badly need this book.

The century of proud progress that marked the 1900s placed medicine securely on its proper scientific platform. Unparalleled growth in subject matter expertise brought to the bedside the benefits of pharmacy, surgery, diagnostic tests, and images in accelerating frequency, and that progress continues. The engine of those gains has been largely the wedding of clinical sciences with other sciences: molecular biology, physics, material sciences, and genetics, for example. The application of new knowledge gained new footing in the later decades of the twentieth century, thanks to deep interactions between medicine and statistics, epidemiology, decision analysis, and emerging evaluative methods of clinical epidemiology. In public policy and care design, econometrics and psychology also gained footholds, with the landmark Rand Health Insurance Experiment ushering in a new era of health services research.

The pattern can be interpreted thus—health care has made progress on two routes—within disciplines and at the intersection of disciplines. Both forms of progress have mattered a great deal, but anyone familiar with these intellectual advances knows that in many ways the development of science on the second route—at intersections—has been the slower and more difficult of the two. To bring molecular epidemiology, statistics, and economics, for example, into the service of health care has required vision, strong

leadership, and a willingness to take risks. Bridging between intellectual pursuits previously unfamiliar with each other requires
translation, patience, an attitude of respect among strangers, and
foundations and other funders willing to offer some venture capital
to the meeting places.

I recall clearly that I first met Professor Pliskin, one of the
authors of this book, under the auspices of then-Dean of the Harvard School of Public Health, Howard Hiatt, who must rank in any
accurate health care history as one of the most courageous and successful intersection builders of our time. Although his formal background had been deeply rooted in classical research in clinical
oncology and molecular biology, by the 1950s well-honored terrain
for formal research, Hiatt had come to feel that progress for health
care as a system—one deeply troubled by defects, excessive cost,
irrational clinical practices, and most urgently, social inequality—
would depend on new interactions between health care knowledge
and other domains of knowledge that, until then, had not had much
to do with clinical care. At the Harvard School of Public Health,
Hiatt created a new "Center for the Evaluation of Clinical Practices" and attracted the interest and attention of some young and
some not-so-young mavericks, some of the stature of Professors Fred
Mosteller, Benjamin Barnes, and Howard Frazier, and others who
were still finding their way into their academic niches, such as Mil-
ton Weinstein, Harvey Fineberg, Duncan Neuhauser, Shan Cretin,
Emmett Keeler, Mark Rosenberg, and me. Joe Pliskin, ready and
able to try to forge new links between operations research and
health care, was soon interacting with us.

The new center and its senior sponsors cut the risks of explor-
ing new terrain together, but not quite to zero. It still took a mod-
icum of risk taking for young statisticians or economists to migrate
away from their disciplinary departments enough to work steadily
and productively with young clinicians equally willing to engage in
research that was hard to explain to their clinically based colleagues.
But it was fun enough to thrive, and from that era at Harvard and

elsewhere came the foundations of a new wave of clinical epidemiology, cost-effectiveness analysis, decision analysis, and health services research that matured fully in the few decades that followed.

One such intersection, however, did not, in my opinion, flourish as it should have. For reasons unclear to me, operations management—the types of quantitative and systems methods so ably explored in this book—did not find the traction in health care that other, related sciences—economics, statistics, and even psychometrics—more rapidly did. As a result, we have today widespread use of valuable psychometric surveys (like the SF-32 and its progeny), widespread commitment to, or at least awareness of, evidence-based medicine, and strong centers of health economics around the United States. The equivalent realization regarding operations management and its related disciplines—that these hold the seeds of crucial understandings and a foundation for change—did not then fully blossom.

Luckily, systems scientists like Ronen and Pliskin, absolutely expert in their disciplines and unwilling to give up their firm interest in health care, continued to pursue their mastery of their fields and their explorations of how health care could benefit. Equally important, new waves of theorists in systems science advanced their basic work and began to explain their rather complex insights in ways that less technically proficient communities could understand: Goldratt, Senge, and others.

Meanwhile, health care has continued to advance on many fronts but to get into deeper and deeper trouble on others. Soaring costs, fragmentation of care, discontinuity, and a growing sense of frustration in the workforce have become symptoms not only in the United States but in almost all developed nations. These authors had originally subtitled their book "Doing More with the Same Resources," and that, exactly, is the heart of the matter that faces almost all health care systems and organizations as the twenty-first century gains momentum.

And it is the disciplines they have mastered and present here that have the greatest possible future leverage on that issue. The concepts we need in health care to "do more with the same resources" are not simple. To explain them to people like me takes the elegance of thinking that Ronen and Pliskin have refined in decades of teaching. But the news is good: the concepts are mature, the teachers are in hand, and the need has crested. It will take only one more step—a giant one, but not impossible—for health care leaders to recognize that, as responsible clinical care required their interest in and use of evaluative clinical sciences in recent times, so will the proper and prudent design of the systems they must now create require their interest in and use of the very best of modern systems sciences—ideas like the theory of constraints, the focus on cycle times, and totally new views of waste and efficiency as presented in this book. Ideas whose time has come are delivered here by teachers ready to help us meet them. One must not underestimate the daunting managerial challenges that the needed changes will bring with them, but the potential payoff is immense.

My close colleague and friend Tom Nolan, a master systems thinker himself, has spoken for several years of the need to "dignify" systems sciences in health care so that we can take advantage of them on behalf of patients and communities. Interested leaders will find no resource to study modern systems theories more dignified or comprehensible than this one. It is time to use what they know.

Donald M. Berwick

To our families

Preface

How can a hospital successfully reduce the response time in the emergency department by 40 percent and at the same time increase the clinical quality, all this using existing resources?

How can one increase the throughput of the operating room by 20 percent using the same resources?

Why do traditional cost-accounting methods prevent hospitals and health maintenance organizations (HMOs) from making better managerial decisions in pricing, costing, investment justification, and make-or-buy decisions, and what are the alternatives for better decision making?

Why do performance measures sometimes undermine value creation?

How can the removal of inexpensive bottlenecks easily increase throughput, reduce response time, and increase quality?

Why do adding more personnel and making more capital investment usually fail to lead to improvement of health care organizations?

These topics and more are the theme of this book on managing health care organizations. The book should be of value to all executive and managerial personnel in every health care organization, including hospitals, HMOs, laboratories, ministries of health, clinics, health insurance departments, and government agencies. It provides practical knowledge and tools for people in managerial as well as staff positions. Moreover, this book will be equally useful for other nonprofit and for-profit organizations, in every sector, public or private, service or industry.

The main theme of the book is that one can do *much more* with the *same resources* in terms of throughput, response time, and quality by using practical tools and techniques. It provides a systemic view and touches on issues of performance measures, operations management, quality, cost accounting, pricing, and above all, value creation and value enhancement. We hope that on reading the book, every person within a health care organization will be able to implement immediate actions resulting in improvement in most performance measures of the organization.

Various chapters present simple tools for more effective management. These tools are accompanied by dozens of real-world examples of their successful use. Chapter 18 helps to identify value drivers and guide decision makers on *where* and *when* to implement various components of value creation. The *how* is highlighted in the specific preceding chapters. Chapter 19 presents an integrative approach that uses many of the simple tools presented in the book through a real-world case study of a major public hospital. The final chapter enables managers to identify and deal first with the most important and easily implementable topics.

The book includes the use of methods such as the theory of constraints that yield fast improvement in systems such as operating rooms and emergency departments. The book demonstrates how simple tools like the focusing table, the focusing matrix, the complete kit concept, and Pareto analysis can increase throughput, reduce response time, and create value in the health care industry.

Based on our vast experience in improving health care systems and surveying the most recent improvements in dozens of organizations, wards, and clinics, the use of the methods can increase throughput in places like operating rooms by 10 to 20 percent and reduce response time in places like emergency departments and clinics by 20 to 40 percent while only using existing resources.

Naturally, this book is also intended to be a text and reference in teaching management of health care organizations, especially operations management in health care and public health programs, both for graduate and undergraduate students. It will also be relevant to related fields such as social work, psychology, and all allied health professions.

The book is based on our own extensive experience in using and successfully implementing all components presented in the book in health care settings. It also reflects our rich teaching experience with managers and students in various settings such as master of business administration (M.B.A.) programs, executive M.B.A. programs, health care management programs, and schools of public health. Our experience encompasses Harvard University (School of Public Health), Columbia University (Graduate School of Business), New York University (Stern School of Business), Tel Aviv University (Faculty of Management), Boston University (School of Management), Ben Gurion University of the Negev (Faculty of Health Sciences, School of Management), in various Kellogg programs (Northwestern University) throughout the world, and in SDA-Bocconi University in Milan, Italy. We plan to use this book as the only textbook in our courses.

Thousands of executives and students were exposed to these methods over the past decade by actively implementing the methods described in the book, taking our courses, or participating in our workshops. Many successful implementations occurred as a result of this exposure. We have led projects where the methods were successfully implemented and achieved both short- and long-term results. Our book presents many case studies and real-world applications that had a strong positive impact in many organizations.

Our approach is applications oriented using new managerial approaches. On the one hand, it is not the typical quantitative operations management book, and on the other hand, it is not an organizational behavior one. It is mission or business oriented (or both), targeted to achieve immediate and substantial improvements in health care organizations.

We would like to acknowledge the valuable contributions of Shany Karmy, Sarah Miller, and Gali Ronen.

About the Authors

BOAZ RONEN is professor of technology management at Tel Aviv University, Faculty of Management, the Leon Recanati Graduate School of Business Administration. He holds a bachelor of science degree in electronics engineering from the Technion, Haifa, Israel, and a master of science degree and a doctorate in business administration from Tel Aviv University, Faculty of Management. Before his academic career, he worked more than ten years in the high-tech industry. His main areas of interest are focused on firms' value enhancement and improving health care organizations. In his work, he combines value creation, management of technology, the strategic and tactical aspects of the theory of constraints (TOC), and advanced management philosophies.

Ronen has provided consultation services for numerous corporations, health care organizations, and government agencies worldwide. During the past twenty years, Ronen has been leading a team that successfully implemented focused management, TOC, and advanced management practices of value creation in dozens of industrial, hi-tech, information technology, health care, and service organizations.

Ronen teaches in the E.M.B.A. and M.B.A. programs at Tel Aviv University. He has been commended numerous times and received the Rectors' Award for outstanding teaching. He was also a visiting professor at the schools of business of New York University;

Columbia University; the Kellogg-Bangkok program in Bangkok, Thailand; Stevens Institute of Technology; and SDA-Bocconi in Milan, Italy. He has published over one hundred articles in leading academic and professional journals and coauthored three books on value creation, focused management, managerial decision making, and cost accounting.

JOSEPH S. PLISKIN is the Sidney Liswood Professor of Health Care Management at Ben Gurion University of the Negev. He is a member of the Department of Industrial Engineering and Management and of the Department of Health Systems Management, where he is the current chair. Pliskin also has an appointment as an adjunct professor at the Department of Health Policy and Management at the Harvard School of Public Health. He also has a long-term teaching involvement at the School of Management at Boston University.

Pliskin received his bachelor of science degree in mathematics and statistics from the Hebrew University in Jerusalem (1969) and his master's (1970) and doctoral (1974) degrees in applied mathematics (operations research) from Harvard University.

Pliskin's research interests focus on clinical decision making, operations management in health care organizations, cost-benefit and cost-effectiveness analysis in health and medicine, technology assessment, utility theory, and decision analysis.

He has published extensively on issues relating to end-stage renal disease, heart disease, Down syndrome, technology assessment, and methodological issues in decision analysis. He is a coauthor of the book *Decision Making in Health and Medicine: Integrating Evidence and Values* (Cambridge University Press, 2001).

SHIMEON PASS is an expert in applying the philosophy and tools of the focused management methodology and theory of constraints (TOC) in high technology, industrial, service, retail, and nonprofit organizations. As an executive at IBM, he specialized in the implementation of advanced managerial methods to enterprise information systems. He is now specializing in applying focused manage-ment and TOC practices in the management of research and devel-opment organizations and project management. His papers on value creation and performance improvement have been published in leading practice and academic journals.

Focused Operations Management for Health Services Organizations

Part I

The Dynamic Health Care Management Environment

The Modern Health Care and Business Environment

Objective

- Why are new managerial approaches needed?

For more than twenty years, the health care systems of most western countries have been faced with the challenge of dealing with massive increases in health care costs in real terms and as a percentage of their gross national products. As a result, they have been obliged to cut expenses in other sectors to provide their people with a reasonable health care system. Classical breakdowns of health care system costs can be shown in either the supply part or the demand part.

During the past two decades, the business environment in many sectors has been characterized by rapid changes. The main revolution has been the transition from a "sellers' market" to a "buyers' market." The *sellers' market,* which was common in the past, refers to a somewhat monopolistic business environment where the supplier or service provider dictates the dimensions of a venture:

- Price: usually determined by a "cost-plus" approach where the customer is charged the full costs of the services rendered plus a "reasonable profit"

- Response time: "We are doing our best, and we are really trying"

- Quality: "We are doing the best we can under the circumstances"

- Performance: "We know better than the customers what they need. We are the professionals"

From a Sellers' Market to a Buyers' Market

Today's business environment is that of a buyers' market. This trend is the result of international revolutions and macroeconomic, technological, political, and social changes. This environment is characterized by

- Globalization of the world economy

- Fierce competition among organizations within and across countries

- Global excess capacities in production, services, and in some areas of development

- Use of new managerial approaches

- Availability and accessibility of data and knowledge

- Cheap and rapid communication

- Timely availability of materials and services

- Ease of global travel and conveyance

- Adoption of advanced technologies for production and development

- Extensive use of advanced computers and information systems

- Extensive use of communications and information technology

- Shortened life cycles of products and services

- Democratization and customer empowerment

Globalization: The Small Global Village

The world is gradually becoming a *world without borders*. In most world regions, particularly in the western countries, one can travel freely without the need for entry visas. Similarly, customs and tariffs on goods transferred across borders have been reduced or totally eliminated. Travel between countries is easy, fast, and cheap, whether it be people, merchandise, or materials.

In the past decade, we have witnessed a trend in the formation of *multinational firms*. Successful companies acquire partial or full ownership of firms in other countries, thus obtaining the advantage of access to additional markets and diversification of the product line of the parent company. Firms engage in international cooperation with foreign firms, resulting in mutual benefits. The world has excess capacity in production and services, and it is essential to find additional market channels and better congruence with customers of the various world markets.

Communication has become global. If we examine television programs, radio broadcasts, and the written media, it seems that many of the programs and their information are transportable "as is" to other parts of the world. People in remote areas watch, for better or worse, the same TV programs, laugh at the same jokes, and are exposed to messages of democracy and an open world.

The globalization trend is not coincidental. It is strongly affected by the end of global wars and the opening of borders, resulting in a shift of resources from military industries to civilian ones, including such services as health care and education, as well as privatization of economic activity. The world has opened up, and we

witness a desire for individual and social welfare, customer empowerment, and awareness of environmental quality. The enhanced
openness has made technological and managerial knowledge acces-
sible to all.

> In a large public hospital, waiting times in the emergency department
> were excessive. Management methods were changed, resulting in a
> 30 percent reduction in patient waiting times; the clinical quality did
> not decrease (and may have actually improved), and patient satis-
> faction from service quality improved. All this was achieved without
> any investment of money, personnel, or equipment by using existing
> information systems and resources and simply by changing man-
> agerial approaches. This hospital is using state-of-the-art telemedi-
> cine technology with global connections for transferring imaging
> information, receiving second opinions, and so forth. There is also an
> increase in the number of out-of-country patients who are accessing
> this hospital, both physically and virtually through telemedicine.

In a buyers' market, the customer determines the following:

• *Price*: determined by the market. Superior quality, unusual features, or performance can usually improve the price by 10 to 15 percent. The manufacturer or service provider must adjust to market
prices to survive. Customers are not interested in how much a service costs the producer or service provider. The market dictates the
price, leaving the producer or provider with the cruel choice of
adjusting to market prices or disappearing.

• *Response time*: determined by the response time of the best in
the market. For example, in the market of film and photo developing, once the one-hour developing emerged, stores with a lead time
of a full day had no chance of surviving.

• *Quality*: determined by the best quality existing in the market. For example: automobiles and electronic equipment are compared with Japanese products that provide the standard for quality.

Even lower prices cannot provide market survival for those who do not perform to standards.

- *Performance*: the customers determine their wishes and needs.

The process of globalization and the shift from a sellers' to a buyers' market also caused shareholders to put pressure on management. Executives, especially in firms with international components, must be evaluated by different criteria than in the past. They deal with shareholders who will not accept excuses, know alternative solutions to problems, and can recommend new managerial approaches and up-to-date managerial standards. Globalization and strong competition result in many firms coping with survival.

In not-for-profit organizations, including government agencies and hospitals, recent years have brought *increased demand* for services on the one hand and *budget reduction* on the other. This situation results in higher pressures on management. Using new managerial approaches and philosophies enables managers to extract from these organizations additional output without increasing resources. For example, in one major hospital, operating room output has increased by 20 percent with the same personnel and with better clinical and service quality.

A similar situation exists in the health care market, characterized by the following features:

- Customers demand more.

- Customers have more and better information.

- Technologies (equipment, medications, devices, and procedures) develop rapidly while budget growth cannot keep pace.

- People have longer life expectancies.

This situation can be nicely described by the "scissors diagram" of Figure 1.1, which shows budgets declining in time and the

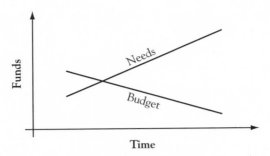

Figure 1.1. "Scissors Diagram" of Needs Versus Budget.

demand for technology, drugs, and pressure to perform increasing the demands on the system.

The Remedy: Adoption of New Managerial Approaches

Advanced technology, professional personnel, and powerful information systems do not guarantee survival in a highly competitive market. They are perhaps necessary or supportive conditions but definitely not sufficient. The main determinant in the ability to survive competition is the adoption of advanced managerial approaches that are compatible with the new business environment.

In recent years, such new approaches have been developed and successfully implemented in many organizations. In many instances, managerial decision making has changed. The foundation for the development of these new approaches is the desire to be compatible with a new business reality and to engage relevant value drivers to improve and enhance the value of these organizations.

Management teams of most organizations have come to realize that to succeed in the global competitive environment, it is not enough to revert to technological innovation or to use cheaper resources and materials. It is essential to manage differently. The new managerial approaches result in enhancing the value of the organization.

Value enhancement: Increasing the value of an organization to its owners, its workers, and the community.

The new managerial approaches have several characteristics:

- They are based on common sense.

- These approaches evolved out of practice; only later did they receive academic and scientific validation.

- They are simple and use the KISS ("keep it simple, stupid") approach.

- They break down the myth of the input-output model.

The input-output myth (see Figure 1.2) implies: "If we want to increase system outputs, we must increase inputs." For example, if we want to increase patient volume in a clinic by 20 percent, we may request more input in the form of personnel, space, advertising, and the like. If we want to decrease waiting time for patients, we again may request more personnel and equipment. The modern managerial approaches show that this myth can be broken. We can *increase output* without increasing input by changing the managerial approach. Evidence for better management of *existing resources* can

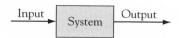

Figure 1.2. The Input-Output Model.

be found in Mabin and Balderstone (2000) and in Coman, Koller, and Ronen (1996). As will be seen in the following chapters, an additional managerial input has been added—that is, a different managerial approach.

Chapter Summary

The world has become a small village with global competition. The market faced by organizations is not just the region or the country in which they operate but the whole world. On the one hand, this creates a threat from organizations outside the country, but on the other hand, it opens opportunities to penetrate huge outside markets. Management has become more difficult and more demanding in light of fierce competition, the increasing complexity and diversity of products and services, and the need to implement advanced technology. Past achievements are becoming obsolete as a result of competitors' improvements. An organization that does not improve will be driven out of the market. Technology, skilled personnel, and information systems are necessary but not sufficient conditions for survival. In addition, there must be the important component of managerial approaches that are congruent with the competitive environment of today.

Not-for-profit organizations, hospitals, government agencies, and others face increased demand for their service while needing to contain costs. Implementation of new managerial approaches will improve their performance.

The objectives of management are to enhance the value of the firm (in business firms) or to improve organizational performance (in task-oriented and not-for-profit organizations). Many organizations are fighting for their survival. They need to identify relevant value drivers and improve them using innovative approaches based on common sense. The bottom line of these approaches is "doing more with what you have."

2

Principles of Management in a Dynamic Environment

- Why most health care organizations resort to suboptimization, and how a global view can avoid this

- Why the "optimizer" approach may interfere with health care organizations achieving their goals and how the "satisficer" approach is an answer

- Why focused management is needed

What Is a System?

A system is a collection of interconnected components acting together toward a common goal. It is a complex and *holistic* entity. It can be a biological system, an engineering system, or an organizational system (business, goal oriented, or not for profit). A system has a *goal* that drives its activity. The overall goal generates defined *quantitative objectives* that must be achieved and *performance measures* that enable management or owners to exercise control and judge whether they are on the right track to achieve the goal. The system has boundaries within the environment it operates. The system consists of *subunits* with *hierarchy* and *interaction*. The system has a *process* that *converts* the *input* it receives from the environment into *output* that the environment receives from the system. Some organizational systems have a *feedback* process by which the system corrects its activity and adjusts itself to environmental changes (see Figure 2.1).

W. Edwards Deming (1986), one of the pioneers of quality management, is responsible for the change in the modern perception of the organizational system. He emphasizes the people in the system, and he includes suppliers and customers within the system definition. Including suppliers and customers indicates that they are partners of the effective operation of the system. Hence, without a full dialogue between the system and its customers on the one hand and between the system and its suppliers on the other, the system's performance cannot be improved. Without such a dialogue, the system cannot comply with its customers' needs and will not receive from its suppliers adequate answers for its needs. This modern outlook is depicted in Figure 2.2.

Goldratt and Cox (1992) added an important layer to system theory by proposing to simplify the way we perceive the system and to focus on its constraints.

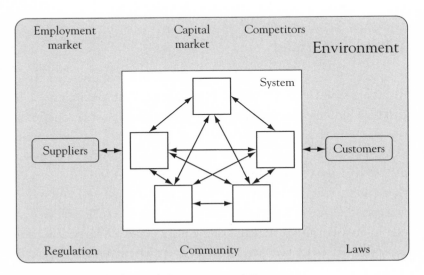

Figure 2.1. A Traditional Organizational System.

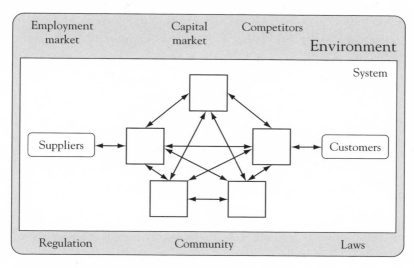

Figure 2.2. A Modern Organizational System.

The performance of the whole system depends on a few factors, designated as the *system constraints* (see Chapter 4). Thus, in a hospital, for example, the operating rooms (ORs) are usually the system constraints (the bottlenecks). The performance of such a system depends mainly on the efficiency and effectiveness of the bottleneck. This simplification, along with the focusing approach, helps to better understand the system and improve it.

System Optimization and Suboptimization

A major managerial failure emanates from the approach that "if every subunit in the system will operate optimally, then the whole system will function optimally." However, an organization in which every subunit is striving to improve performance without examining interaction with other subunits, or without examining the relation between these activities and the overall objectives and performance of the whole organization, may find itself with adverse effects on organizational performance. This phenomenon is referred to as suboptimization or local optimization. This phenomenon results from interaction among subsystems, from improper performance measures, or from the fact that a local objective function of a subsystem is not congruent with the overall objective function of the organization.

Suboptimization of a system: separate optimization of every subsystem, which results in *underutilization* of the performance potential of the whole system and may result in a deterioration of overall performance.

The purchasing department in a hospital was measured by purchasing costs and discounts obtained from suppliers. The desire to minimize costs drove purchasing managers to buy inferior-quality products. The poor quality caused clinical and service failures and an increase in repeated hospitalizations of many patients. Overall, the hospital's performance was compromised.

In a large hospital's surgical ward, most attention was given to optimizing performance and scheduling in the ORs. At the same time, the ward suffered from many cases of infections, thus negatively affecting the hospital's performance and achievement of goals.

Suboptimization is usually caused by a local focus of the sub-organization, by measuring those suborganizations in a way that local improvements do not necessarily improve the organization as a whole, or using a local objective function that is not congruent with the overall objective function of the organization.

The "Satisficer" Versus the "Optimizer"

Nobel laureate H. A. Simon recognized many years ago a managerial situation that causes decision-making hardship, and his approach revolutionized management. Simon (1957) claimed that executives, engineers, and decision makers are trying to become optimizers while making decisions.

Optimizer: A decision maker who wants to make the *best possible decision* without consideration of time constraints.

To achieve the best possible decision, one must generate all the alternatives, gather all the information, and build a model that will evaluate the alternatives and choose the best one. All this requires time, effort, and money. In the real world, there is no limit to the number of alternatives one can evaluate. We are all familiar with the situation where a group of executives and professionals gathers and someone says that "we have not examined all the possibilities." With every variety of alternatives, someone will always be able to claim that more time should be invested in examining additional options.

Information retrieval may not be easy. If it is mostly outside the organization, it also costs money. In addition, the information that is available inside the organization is not error- or bias-free. Hence, decision makers will never have all the needed information on hand to evaluate every alternative.

Building the optimal model to evaluate alternatives is also time- and labor-intensive. Finding an optimal solution to a problem necessitates much preparation: defining all the decision variables, collecting all the relevant data (time studies, demand, labor resources, suppliers, customers, quantities, costs, batch sizes, delivery times, orders, inventory, and so forth), building a model that will describe the real situation, identifying optimization and calculation methods, and obtaining software and hardware to perform the optimization.

The perfect solution sought by the optimizer may bring about a better decision, but it may come too late. In a dynamic world, changes are frequent, and it is of utmost importance to make timely decisions that respond to market situations. Thus, optimal solutions, even if attainable, become *irrelevant* if they are obsolete—that is, the environment and the competition have changed, as have prices, laws, and regulations. Trying to behave as an optimizer results in "analysis paralysis." In the medical world, "until the doctors decide, the patient will die."

Simon (1957) proposes an alternative approach and suggests that decision makers behave as "satisficers"—that is, that they aspire to reach a satisfactory solution and not necessarily a perfect (or optimal) one.

Satisficer: A decision maker who is *satisfied* with a reasonable solution that will significantly improve the system and does not look for the optimal solution.

The satisficer sets a *level of aspiration*, a threshold that he or she aspires to achieve (see Figure 2.3). The objective is not to maximize or minimize some performance measure but to achieve a solution that will improve the measure beyond the predefined level of aspiration. Satisficers need not examine all the alternatives. They can examine some of them until they find one that brings them over the threshold. Once the level of aspiration has been met, the satisficer may set a new aspiration level. This iterative process is one of con-

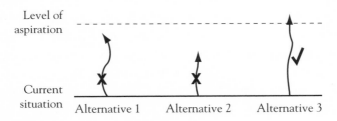

Figure 2.3. The Satisficer's Approach.

tinued organizational improvement. This approach is time efficient. Satisficers do not waste precious time searching for the ultimate solution. They quickly identify steps that may significantly improve their current situation.

A satisficer achieves excellence by complying with two principles:

1. Set a high enough level of aspiration that is compatible with market conditions, competition, or investor expectations.
2. Adopt an approach of continuous improvement.

The level of aspiration is set according to investor expectations for return on investment, the performance of the best competitor, market conditions, business opportunities, necessary conditions for survival, and the like. Continuous improvement is essential for further value enhancement of a firm. A one-time improvement gives the firm a temporary relative advantage over competitors. Without a process of continuous improvement, this relative advantage will be lost.

Whereas the optimizer uses optimization techniques, the satisficer uses heuristics, which are decision rules that are not necessarily optimal but yield improvement (see Figure 2.4).

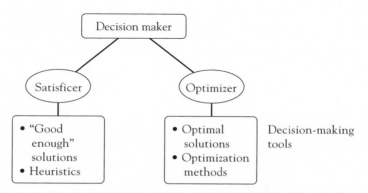

Figure 2.4. Decision-Making Process: Optimizer Versus Satisficer.

A hospital wanted to computerize patient records. A consulting firm was hired to analyze the system and its needs and to design and implement a new computer system. The process took six years. After an additional two years, the technology changed, making the system obsolete. A competing hospital in the same city adopted a computerized patient record system used in other hospitals. The system was installed and adapted to the specific needs of the hospital. Within one year, the system was operating successfully, with concurrent development for more specific needs. The first hospital tried to find the optimal solution and was without a record system for six years while incurring high development and consulting costs. The competitor settled for some satisfactory level of aspiration and had a satisfactory working system within a year at considerably lower cost.

The managerial approaches presented in this book are based on the satisfier approach and on heuristics, hence their suitability for the dynamic managerial environment of today. We are not providing problem-free "perfect" solutions. However, there is no doubt that the suggested solutions are good and bring about significant improvement. On a philosophical level, the organization need not function perfectly; it only needs to perform better than its competitors.

The optimizer approach may generate better solutions to some problems. However, the assortment of approaches and solutions presented in this book have passed market and reality tests and are ready for immediate implementation. A common wisdom among engineers and software professionals is that "The enemy of 'good' is 'better.'"

Elements of Focused Management

To survive the fierce competition of today, an organization must continuously enhance its value and improve performance: do more with the same resources. Organizational performance can be enhanced by improving its value drivers using appropriate managerial approaches. Integrating managerial approaches and adapting their mix to organizational culture and environment improve the chances for better performance and value enhancement. The following managerial approaches characterize focused management:

- Constraint management using the theory of constraints

- Approaches to reduce response time

- The "compete kit" concept

- New approaches for measurement and control

- The global decision-making three-stage model for making decisions about pricing, transfer prices, and the like

- Approaches for formulating an operational business strategy

- The value-focused management approach

- Methods for quality improvement and process control

All these approaches will be discussed in subsequent chapters.

Focused management thrives on improving organizational performance by employing and adapting a mix of managerial approaches for every organization and identifying the relevant value drivers and focusing on them.

Value drivers: Performance variables whose improvement will significantly increase the value of a business firm or significantly increase the performance measures of a not-for-profit organization.

In a business organization (see Chapter 18), the value is defined as the discounted cash flow. The following are examples of possible value drivers:

- Increased contribution from sales

- Reduced time to market in developing products and services

- Increased throughput of operations and development activities in the organization

- Strategic focus

- Improved quality

Experience (including numerous organizations with whom we were involved) demonstrates that using a variety of managerial approaches and adapting them to specific needs bring significant performance improvements.

Focused Management Triangle

The focused management triangle (see Figure 2.5) reflects the following basic principles of focused management: a global system view, focusing on essentials, and using simple tools.

A Global System View

Appropriate management should consider the effect of a current decision on the whole system and not only on the single unit or subsystem. A global system view reduces organizational suboptimization.

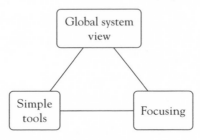

Figure 2.5. Focused Management Triangle.

Global vision requires expanding the system approach in two dimensions: the scope and the time frame.

Expanding the Scope of the System

In the decision-making process, every manager of a subsystem must evaluate everything from a global perspective to avoid suboptimization.

In a private hospital, there was an effort to increase OR capacity. Throughput increased, but the number of patients requiring surgery did not. When expanding to view the larger system, it was discovered that the recovery rooms did not have sufficient capacity to contain the increased capacity of the ORs.

A high-tech medical imaging firm developed a superior product with unique and innovative performance. On completion of the prototype, it was discovered that they used components that are difficult to purchase, production is difficult, and the dimensions of the packaging exceeded what major customers want. Performance is part of the system outlook. If decisions had been made from a global perspective, it would have been clear that it was necessary to examine, as early as possible, customer requirements, performance, response times, productivity, marketing, and sales.

In a certain cellular phone company, sales personnel were rewarded by the number of new subscribers they brought in. The sales force heavily recruited customers who contributed little to profit and also presented high risk in bill payment. This performance measure also led to selling new lines to existing customers with the request to silence their existing lines. They were rewarded for generating new lines that in fact did not generate any new call volume. The bottom-line result was increased costs to the company without the addition of real sales.

Expanding the Time Frame

A proper process of development considers the total life cycle of a product and includes issues of production, maintenance, checking, failure modes, and more. Expansion within time emphasizes the concept of "life-cycle cost." When purchasing materials and components or when choosing and buying equipment, one must globally evaluate the life-cycle cost of the component, product, or equipment to make better decisions for the whole system. In the decision-making process, a manager must consider not only short-term but also medium- and long-term issues.

One of the branches of a health agency prepared medical emergency kits. Every item in the kit was chosen from a cost-effectiveness perspective. Within a short time, it was learned that one of the items, a tourniquet, had a shelf life of one year, whereas all other items had a shelf life of four years. The tourniquet was plastic and was cheap (2 cents each). This situation required refreshing the kit every year with a new tourniquet, which necessitated disassembling the whole kit and then reassembling. This annual maintenance was costly. After some consideration, it was decided to purchase a more expensive high-quality elastic tourniquet with a shelf life of four years. This resulted in a longer shelf life of the whole kit and drastically reduced maintenance costs. The original approach looked at the short-term (low) purchasing costs without considering the longer life-cycle cost of the whole kit.

A hospital was considering the purchase of a computed tomographic scanner. There were price differences in the quotations with no apparent differences in performance. The temptation was to purchase the cheapest unit. When the entire life-cycle cost was evaluated, the decision switched to buying the scanner with the lowest life-cycle cost, which turned out to be the one with the most expensive initial price. In subsequent purchases, suppliers were required to provide full life-cycle figures.

A large public hospital received a donation to build an additional, high-class building. The building was constructed and is now functioning. However, it is clear to management that the maintenance costs are excessively high and that the hospital will not be able to maintain the building beyond its first few years.

A health maintenance organization (HMO) started using a global view in the time dimension, which resulted in a shift to invest more in disease prevention than in disease treatment. This solution led to better health for the insured customers and a drastic reduction in costs as a result of decreased utilization of medical services. The HMO recommended free flu immunizations to members older than fifty-five. They initiated a measurement process of the percentage vaccinated in each clinic and provided feedback to the primary care physicians. The number of pneumonia hospitalizations during that year dropped significantly when compared with previous years.

It is obvious that every system is a subsystem of a larger system. As such, it is vulnerable to suboptimization. Management must *reduce* suboptimizations by exposing others to their dangers and working together to avoid them.

Focusing on Essentials

Executives and managers' time is scarce. Organizations are continually struggling with daily crises, and the time devoted to "extinguishing fires" does not leave room for change and improvement. Even for routine operations, it is difficult to find the time to deal with all issues. However, every issue that management wants to advance will get priority and consideration and will frequently be implemented. Hence, management's focus on a few important topics will yield significant improvement.

Focusing on essentials is one principle of successful management. The problems and tasks of a manager can be classified into four types, based on the Pareto principle (see Chapter 3). This classification is presented in Figure 2.6.

- Type A problems: These are few but important; *solving them will contribute much to the organization.* They are usually difficult problems that require time and management resources.

- Type B problems: These represent several problems with medium importance; solving them will contribute to the organization.

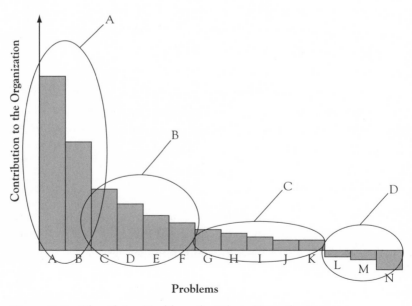

Figure 2.6. Classifying Problems by Their Contribution to the Organization.

- Type C problems: Many routine problems are easy to deal with; solving them will contribute little.

- Type D problems: A large collection of problems are easy to deal with, but spending time on them will bring negative utility by taking up valuable management time that could have been used in solving important problems.

Many executives spend much of their time dealing with type C problems rather than type A. This happens when the "urgent" (C) pushes aside the "important" (A). Management must *focus on type A problems of the organization*. Managers must focus on those issues where a small effort can have a large effect on improving organizational performance. As we shall see in the next chapters, managers must focus on system constraints, bottlenecks, critical tasks in projects, risk factors, and more. There is a need for a uniform language, determination, and managerial maturity to shift attention to what is important.

Because of the complexity of management and the obstacles facing managers, they do not have more than 10 to 15 percent of their time to deal with essentials and improve value drivers whose outcomes will be realized only several months down the road. Therefore, they must set aside what little time remains to deal with the *real* problems, thus enhancing organizational value and improving performance.

The world of management is complex and complicated. But as we shall see in future chapters, this world can be made simpler if we focus on a few points whose improvement will improve the system as a whole.

In a large hospital, the purchasing manager realized that the purchasing personnel need not be involved in every purchase. She realized that 70 percent of purchases are for less than $200. She changed policy so that every purchase for less than $200 could be authorized by the manager of every department from a small-purchase budget. This purchase could be made over the phone (from a predetermined list of suppliers who agreed on special prices), leaving the purchasing department time to deal only with large orders. This freed up valuable time of purchasing directors to deal with other important issues.

Later chapters examine various focus areas: type A items using Pareto analysis, constraints and bottlenecks, the "critical chain" in project management, and root problems in an organization.

Simple Tools

Complex managerial tools are not usually used in organizations, and the ones that are used do not significantly contribute to enhancing value. ("What will not be simple will simply not be.") Using such complex managerial tools has not brought remedy to managerial pains. The ensuing chapters present simple tools that can be implanted in various managerial environments: the seven focus stages of management by constraints, the focus stages of the Pareto principle, the focus table and matrix, a focused current reality tree, a conflict-resolution diagram, and additional tools.

Chapter Summary

- Today's business environment is dynamic and difficult to manage.

- The manager faces fierce competition and uncertainty.

- To reach effective decisions, the manager must view the system globally, focus on the essentials, and use simple tools.

- The manager of a subsystem can apply a global system view by considering a *broader* system than the one he or she is heading and by considering a *longer time horizon*.

- Focusing on essentials involves focusing on system constraints, type A items in the Pareto analysis, and the root problems of an organization.

- Implementation of simple tools is successful. The three-stage focusing approach and the focusing table help managers focus on essentials and work more effectively.

- Modern managerial approaches are based on several principles:

  Use the satisficer approach, which wants to achieve a significant improvement and not an endless search for the perfect (optimal) solution.

  Do more with what you have: increase output using existing resources.

  Apply common sense and daily experience.

3

The Pareto Rule, Focusing Table, and Focusing Matrix

Objective

- Know how, when, and why to use the Pareto method, the focusing table, and the focusing matrix

The Pareto Rule

Only a few of the simple principles of management have the ability to contribute enormously through intelligent use. Among these, the Pareto rule deserves special attention and is one of the most important principles of management.

Vilfredo Pareto (1848–1923) was an economist of Italian ancestry who discovered that roughly 20 percent of the population possesses 80 percent of world wealth. This is referred to as the "20-80 rule" or the "principle of the vital few and the trivial many."

Many phenomena in the world of management follow the Pareto rule:

- 20 percent of the patients in a hospital ward consume 80 percent of caregivers' time.

- 20 percent of patients consume 80 percent of medications.

- 20 percent of medications account for 80 percent of pharmaceutical costs.

- 20 percent of laboratory tests account for 80 percent of laboratory costs.

- 20 percent of stores in a supermarket chain account for 80 percent of the chain's profits.

- 20 percent of suppliers provide about 80 percent of the value of products, materials, and components.

- 20 percent of company projects produce about 80 percent of profits.

- 20 percent of hospital inventory items constitute about 80 percent of the total inventory value.

- 20 percent of the sales force is responsible for 80 percent of company sales.

- 20 percent of failure modes in an operating room constitute about 80 percent of all failures in surgery.

- 20 percent of a firm's customers generate 80 percent of the firm's revenues.

In the 1940s, the 20-80 rule was expanded to the three-way classification known today as the ABC classification as follows:

- Group A: 20 percent of phenomenon factors that are responsible for 80 percent of phenomenon outcomes

- Group B: 30 percent of phenomenon factors that are responsible for 10 percent of outcomes

- Group C: 50 percent of phenomenon factors that are responsible for 10 percent of outcomes

For example:

- Group A: 20 percent of patients in a ward account for 80 percent of ward expenses.

- Group B: 30 percent of patients account for 10 percent of expenses.

- Group C: 50 percent of patients account for the remaining 10 percent of expenses.

The Pareto Diagram

A Pareto diagram (see Figure 3.1) visually displays the Pareto rule, enabling the classification and analysis to be better communicated. It is a simple and clear instrument with excellent field experience. The following steps are used to derive the Pareto diagram for a managerial situation:

1. List all the sources of the phenomenon along with their contribution to the situation.

2. Sort the sources by descending order of contribution, from the most to the least.

3. Draw a histogram of all situation sources, as shown in Figure 3.1.

Example: Pareto Analysis of Drug Use in a Hospital

Let us consider the consumption of twelve popular drugs in a hospital ward. The data are presented in Table 3.1. Each drug is evaluated by its monthly costs: that is, the cost of every unit multiplied by the number of units used in a month. Let us now sort Table 3.1 from the drug with the highest dollar cost to the drug with the lowest cost. This is presented in Table 3.2. We are now ready to prepare the Pareto diagram (see Figure 3.2) from Table 3.2.

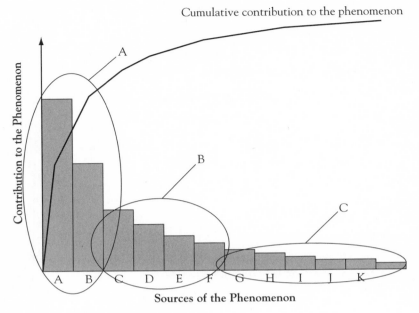

Figure 3.1. Pareto Diagram.

Table 3.1. Drug Use Volume and Costs in a Hospital Ward.

Drug	Cost per Unit ($)	Units Consumed per Month	Total Cost ($ thousands)
A	180	361	65
B	250	160	40
C	950	347	330
D	90	389	35
E	75	267	20
F	560	89	50
G	1,350	11	15
H	650	169	110
I	220	114	25
J	15	1,333	20
K	56	1,518	85
L	150	1,367	205

Table 3.2. Classification by Drug Costs.

Drug	Cost ($ thousands)
C	330
L	205
H	110
K	85
A	65
F	50
B	40
D	35
I	25
E	20
J	20
G	15

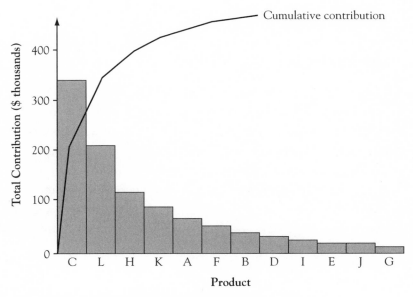

Figure 3.2. Pareto Diagram of Analysis of Drug Costs.

The Pareto analysis as shown in Figure 3.2 brings us to two additional focusing steps: differentiation and appropriate resource allocation.

Building a Pareto Diagram

The following steps are used to build a Pareto diagram:

1. List all sources of a phenomenon. For each source, list the contribution to the phenomenon in the relevant measure (financial, frequency, contribution to response time, downtime, and so forth; see Table 3.1).

2. Rank all sources in descending order from the source whose contribution is the largest to that with the smallest contribution (see Table 3.2).

3. Draw a histogram of the sources where the y axis depicts the contribution such that the height of the bar for each source is proportional to the contribution of that source (see Figure 3.2).

Pareto-Based Focusing Method

Managers use the Pareto rule in all areas of life, some intuitively and some methodically. The Pareto rule is effective and efficient in the presence of resource constraints (also known as a scarce resource or bottleneck), as is discussed in Chapter 4. Managers are frequently the bottlenecks in their system, and the Pareto rule can sort things out. This is also true for sales and marketing personnel, purchasers, and any other scarce resource. The Pareto rule is applicable in areas with resource shortages (bottlenecks), allowing one to devote full attention to all areas.

To effectively apply the Pareto rule, use the following focusing method:

1. *Classification*: Classify the sources of the phenomenon.

2. *Differentiation*: Apply a differential policy.

3. *Resource allocation*: Assign resources appropriately.

Example 1: Applying the Focusing Method in Purchasing

In a large health maintenance organization (HMO), the purchasing personnel in the purchasing department are a system bottleneck. They do not have the time to negotiate successfully with all suppliers and must, therefore, use a focusing method as follows:

1. *Classification:* Purchasers must classify suppliers by the ABC classification described earlier:

   Group A suppliers: The big suppliers are 20 percent of all suppliers and account for 80 percent of the dollar value of all purchases.

   Group B suppliers: The 30 percent medium suppliers account for 10 percent of the total value of purchases.

   Group C suppliers: The small suppliers constitute 50 percent of all suppliers but only 10 percent of purchase value.

2. *Differentiation:* A differential policy must be set for each supplier group:

   For group A suppliers, comprehensive negotiations should be carried out at the beginning of the year, and detailed negotiations on the largest purchasing orders should be carried out throughout the year.

   For group B suppliers, a group of selected suppliers will be chosen, and comparative price follow-up will be done periodically for items purchased from them.

   For group C suppliers, price discounts will be negotiated annually.

3. *Resource allocation:*

Most purchasers' resources should be devoted to negotiations with group A suppliers.

Few resources should be invested in dealing with group B suppliers.

Group C suppliers will be evaluated occasionally.

Note that the above examples related to classification of suppliers or parts by monetary contribution and emphasized that using the method is essential for effective management. It may not always be sufficient to focus on monetary contribution. Occasionally other criteria should be adopted to classify the criticality of items, such as lead time from order of item until delivery; delayed delivery of an item, which can delay production; an item being produced by a single manufacturer; or that shortages in an item can be expected. The purchasing department should, therefore, along with other technical departments, classify items using another Pareto classification that relates to item criticality (see Livne and Ronen, 1990).

Example 2: Applying the Focusing Method in Monitoring Drug Consumption

A large HMO wishes to examine and control the drug consumption of its patients. A Pareto classification was used.

1. *Classification:* Patients were classified according to the monetary value of the drugs they consumed:

Group A patients are the 15 percent of patients who were responsible for 75 percent of the dollar cost of drug consumption.

Group B patients are the 25 percent of patients with moderate drug consumption, which accounts for 15 percent of total drug costs.

Group C patients are the remaining 60 percent of patients who consume only 10 percent of the drugs.

2. *Differentiation:* Applying a different policy for each group:

Group A patients will be evaluated by the medical director of the HMO and the chief pharmacist. Every prescription must be approved by the medical director.

Random sampling of prescriptions for group B patients will be initiated to verify reasonable and cost-effective practice. The sample will cover about 10 percent of prescriptions.

Only 5 percent of patients in group C will be randomly evaluated.

3. *Resource allocation:*

Most cost-containment resources for managing drug consumption will be devoted to group A patients. Only limited resources will be targeted to groups B and C patients.

The Focusing Table and the Focusing Matrix

The focusing table and the focusing matrix are methods that expand the Pareto analysis and include the effort or cost involved in dealing with each factor as well as the benefit. The analysis has two stages:

1. Building the focusing table (also known as the "easy-important table")

2. Building the focusing matrix

Building the Focusing Table

The following example will demonstrate the building of the focusing table:

The emergency department (ED) of a large hospital is considering changing the way it operates. It convenes all people involved in the routine operation of the ED and some top-level executives of the hospital. After many discussions and feedback, they are left with eight suggestions for change and improvement. Every suggestion is assessed according to its importance in being able to bring about improvement, and each suggestion is also assessed according to the ease in time and money of implementing it. Each suggestion is given an importance score ranging from 1 (unimportant) to 5 (very important) and a score for ease of implementation ranging from 1 (very difficult to implement because of many bottlenecks and resources) to 5 (very easy to implement).

Note that the focusing table is an approximation to "specific contribution," which is discussed in Chapter 5. It is clear that if the measures listed in the case example can be adequately quantified, it is better to classify by specific contribution. The focusing table for the ED example is given in Table 3.3.

Generating the Focusing Matrix

Once the focusing table is completed, the focusing matrix is generated (see Figure 3.3). The preferred suggestions are those near the upper right corner of the matrix. Suggestion 5 dominates over all others because it is the most important and the easiest to implement. Between suggestions 3 and 7, there is no dominance relationship, and the decision makers can exercise priorities. The decision makers must choose a set of suggestions to implement and the focusing matrix is an effective tool for making this decision.

The focusing matrix can be useful for the following situations, some of which will be dealt with in the next chapters:

- Choosing among patient case studies to be discussed in morning rounds

- Choosing among projects to be budgeted using a hospital's development fund

Table 3.3. Emergency Department (ED) Focusing Table.

Item Number	Suggestion	Importance[a]	Ease of Implementing[b]
1	Separate ED into surgical and internal wards	4	2
2	Change strategy regarding amount of testing	5	2
3	Open additional imaging room using same personnel	4	5
4	Increase frequency of visits by specialists	4	4
5	Increase frequency of lab workup	5	5
6	Measure average waiting times	4	4
7	Shorten discharge procedure	5	4
8	Redesign admission process	3	3

[a]Scale is 1 (unimportant) to 5 (important).

[b]Scale is 1 (very difficult) to 5 (very easy).

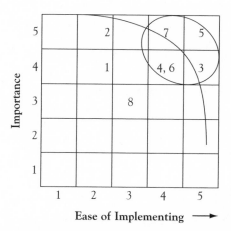

Figure 3.3. Focusing Matrix for the ED Example in Table 3.3.

- Choosing among activities in the process of organizational improvement

Guidelines for Using the Focusing Table and Focusing Matrix

The following guidelines help in using a focusing table and focusing matrix:

1. Make a list of subjects (eight to twelve) to deal with, and arrange them in a focusing table like the example in Table 3.3: number and subject and their importance and ease of implementing.
2. Arrange the subjects in a focusing matrix by importance and ease of implementing, as in Figure 3.3.
3. Choose the subjects for immediate attention. Preference is for subjects in the upper right corner of the matrix, which are both important and easy to implement.

Occasionally it may be wise to even choose subjects that are difficult to implement but whose value is such that they can help improve the system. On the other hand, it may be wise to consider steps that are easily implementable but with little contribution, just to demonstrate quick achievements and results. The eventual choice of subjects is a portfolio choice problem.

Use, Misuse, and Abuse of the Pareto Rule

The Pareto rule is based on several underlying assumptions: independence, importance, equal treatment costs, and use of relevant performance measures.

- *Independence:* The sources of the situation investigated are mutually independent. The assumption of independence is not always valid because some of the causes or sources of a given situation are interdependent. However, even in the presence of such dependence, a Pareto analysis is a good and sufficient first approximation for significant managerial improvement.

• *Constraint:* The sources of a situation relate to a scarce resource (a constraint or a bottleneck). The rationale behind the Pareto rule is the inability to deal with all problems because of resource constraints. Thus, when a resource is a system constraint (see Chapter 4), one must decide what will or will not be done. Naturally, the focus should be on what is most essential for the organization. Hence, Pareto analysis is only relevant in the presence of resource shortages such as budget, personnel, bottleneck time, and the like.

• *Importance:* The severity of the phenomenon is a measure of importance. The assumption of importance is not true in many situations. For example, there are failures with low incidence but with severe consequences because of the damage they cause, and there are frequent failures with negligible damage. Thus, it is recommended to use Pareto analysis where the relevant benefits or damages are on the y axis. This is called an *outcome-based Pareto analysis.*

• *Equal treatment costs:* The effort or costs of treating each source of a situation are equal. It is not true that the efforts and costs needed to deal with a specific factor are the same. There could be a source of importance B that can be dealt with easily and with low cost. Hence, it is better to use the focusing table (easy-important) described earlier in this chapter. The focusing table is actually a two-dimensional Pareto analysis of the difficulty in treating each problem source.

• *Use of relevant performance measures:* The issues for treatment are chosen correctly and will lead to improved system performance. It is not always the case that dealing with each situation requires using measures that are relevant for achieving organizational goals. For example, there are insurance companies that base their decisions on income from premiums ("production") and not on contribution or profit. A market analysis or health insurance agent evaluation based on this nonrelevant production characteristic could result in failure and severe consequences for the insurance company.

Solutions to Failures of Pareto Rule Implementation

When implementing the Pareto rule fails to achieve desired goals, the following criteria should be assured:

- Pareto analysis will be performed only for situations related to scarce resources (see Chapter 4).

- The situation will be measured by performance measures correlated with organizational goals such as contribution, profit, or operational availability.

- When the efforts or costs needed to treat different sources of a situation are not equal, it is wise to resort to using a focusing matrix and focusing table.

Chapter Summary

Pareto analysis is a highly useful tool for managers in every area of management. A manager who does not intensively employ the Pareto rule does not fully utilize its potential. The focusing method is an effective tool in today's complex management world. The method *focuses* the manager on what is important and essential and transforms decision making into a simpler and clearer task.

The use of the focusing method requires a high level of management, especially during the differentiation stage. This stage requires making a variety of simultaneous policy decisions on various levels and the ability to classify various situations for each policy.

Using the Pareto rule and focusing method can greatly assist in managerial decision-making processes. First, it is a tool that differentiates between the important and more important and allows focusing on the most important issues. A Pareto analysis using the focusing method focuses decision makers on a few areas that will require most of their attention. Focusing on group A items or the upper right corner of the focusing matrix allows for an effective use of management time.

This chapter presented some of the nicest, easiest, and simplest tools for focusing, extracting scarce resources, and good communication in an organization.

Part II

Novel Management Approaches

Management by Constraints

The Focusing Steps
of the Theory of Constraints

Objectives

- How to do more with existing resources using the theory of constraints approach

- How to identify the various constraints

Management by constraints is an innovative and effective approach to management developed by Goldratt and Cox (1992). This has been a managerial breakthrough, and in the past fifteen years its use has brought about significant improvements in thousands of organizations worldwide. The seven focusing steps of management by constraints are based on the conceptual foundation of such methods as linear programming (Ronen and Starr, 1990). The method of management by constraints is typical for the satisficer approach (see Chapter 2). It provides satisfactory solutions that bring about significant and rapid improvements in organizational performance.

Management by constraints is based on a seven-step process. The first three of these steps are discussed further in this chapter and the rest in the next chapter.

1. Determine the system's goal.

2. Establish global performance measures.

3. Identify the system constraint.

4. Decide how to exploit the constraint; "break" dummy and policy constraints.

5. Subordinate the rest of the system to the constraint.

6. Elevate and break the constraint.

7. If the constraint is broken, return to step 3. Do not let inertia become a system constraint.

Step 1: Determine the System's Goal

The goal of an organization is of utmost importance because it should guide every decision and action in the organization. Once the goal has been determined, every person in the organization must evaluate every decision or action as to its congruence with this goal. Unfortunately, not enough attention is devoted to this important area.

The goal is something we aspire to but can never achieve: for example, to achieve maximal value, to have zero accidents or zero hospital-based infections. The goal of a business organization is to *increase shareholders' value*. As a first approximation to the real goal of a business organization, one can talk about maximal cash flow or maximum profit over time: simply stated, "making more money now as well as in the future" (Goldratt and Cox, 1992). It is clear that such a goal can sustain itself over time only if the interests of workers, suppliers, customers, and the community are taken into consideration.

In not-for-profit organizations, the goal is determined by the mission of the organization. In such organizations, the goal is usually determined as achieving the maximum of some measure under resource constraints (such as budget). For example, the goal of a public health care organization is to maximize quality medical services provided to its customers, subject to budgetary constraints. Such organizations may have several goals or complex goals. For example, the goals of highway patrol are to prevent accidents and improve traffic flow. The process of defining the goal(s) of not-for-profit organizations is extremely important, even if it may take a long time.

Consider the goals of an emergency department (ED) of a hospital. There could be two approaches to patient management: make a quick decision on admission or discharge, or provide a comprehensive diagnostic workup. These two goals are actually conflicting ones.

While determining the goal of any divisions or departments within an organization, it is important to ensure congruence of the goal with that of the whole organization. The absence of such congruence can easily lead to suboptimization.

The medical division of a large health maintenance organization (HMO) set an objective of providing high-quality medical care. One goal of the HMO was to minimize the life-cycle cost of treating its patients. The goal of the medical division was changed to providing adequate preventive services that will improve overall health and will lead to long-term cost reduction.

The head of a surgical ward in a large hospital decided to introduce a rare and complicated surgical procedure to enhance the hospital's prestige at a time when the main competitor was performing such procedures. The new venture resulted in longer waits for the more standard procedures that yield higher clinical quality to patients and higher profits to the hospital.

Step 2: Establish Global Performance Measures

To be able to evaluate the managerial activity of an organization and determine if it helps achieve the goal, we must decide on global performance measures that are compatible with the goal of the organization. Performance measures of an organization are a guiding compass that point in the direction toward the goal. Relevant measures for a business organization are the *value of the company* (defined as the present value of cash flow) and measures of *economic value added*, described in Chapter 18. Sometimes it is difficult to see the relation between midlevel managerial decisions and measures of cash flow or value enhancement. Thus, there is a need for additional measures.

There is no single perfect performance measure that, despite showing evidence of improvement, will achieve the organizational goal. However, we can define an array of six basic performance measures, each of which measures a different dimension of organizational performance. They are throughput (T), operating expenses (OE), inventory (I), response time (RT), quality (Q), and due-date performance (DDP). These measures are used for managerial control, for rewarding executives and workers, and for supporting decision-making processes. Chapter 13 expands on this topic.

Defining organizational objectives uses organizational performance measures. The organizational objectives are quantitative objectives defined in terms of relevant performance measures. As opposed to the goal, the *objectives* should be defined in a manner that makes them *achievable*.

Step 3: Identify the System Constraint

The philosophy of management by constraints is based on identifying the causes that *halt* the system and *prevent* it from achieving its goal. The concept behind this approach is unique because there is no search for factors that can help improve system performance but rather a search for factors that *restrict* system performance. The relevant question is, What stops the system? or What prevents the system from achieving the goal?

Constraint: Any important factor that prevents an organization from reaching its goal.

Every system has a constraint. There is always something that prevents it from achieving its goal. If there were no constraints, the system would achieve unbounded performance. Experience shows that systems have a *small number of constraints*—a few factors that prevent them from achieving their goals. There are four types of constraints in a managerial system:

- Resource constraint

- Market constraint

- Policy constraint

- Dummy constraint

Resource Constraint

Because the resource constraint is the system constraint, the system cannot achieve its goal. If the capacity of the constraining resource was bigger, it would be possible to increase system throughput and improve the extent of achieving the goal.

Resource constraint (or bottleneck): The most heavily utilized resource such that it cannot perform all its assigned tasks. This is the resource that constrains the performance of the entire system.

Figure 4.1 presents examples of various managerial systems, including a medical one. The framework of a 1–2–3 process can represent a variety of work processes.

In the process depicted in Figure 4.2, every patient must be processed in each of the three departments, beginning with department 1 and ending in department 3. Department 2 is the resource that is the system constraint because it can process only 50 patients per day whereas the market demands processing 300 patients per day. Department 2 is the resource that dictates the throughput of the whole system to be at most 50 patients per day. Departments 1

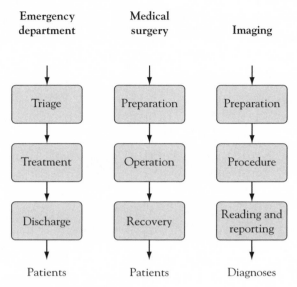

Figure 4.1. System Processes.

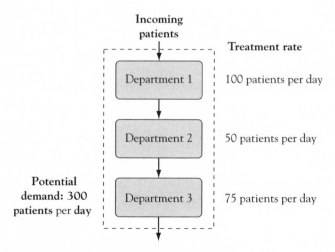

Figure 4.2. A System with a Resource Constraint.

and 3, even though they cannot provide the full daily demand, do not constrain the system throughput and thus are not treated as system constraints.

In the example of Figure 4.2, we say that

- The system has a *resource constraint*.

- Department 2 is the system *bottleneck*.

It should be noted that if we increase the daily capacity of departments 1 and 3, the throughput (capacity) of the whole system will not change. On the other hand, increasing the throughput of department 2 will increase system throughput. The bottleneck, department 2, dictates the throughput for the whole system and should be treated as the organizational "goose that lays golden eggs." A lost hour in the bottleneck is a lost hour for the entire system (Goldratt and Cox, 1992). We should consider the bottleneck as the "money-printing machine" of the organization: the higher its utilization, the higher the throughput of the whole system.

Bottlenecks exist in all areas of life:

- In an operating room (OR) of one hospital, the bottleneck was the surgeon; in another hospital, it was the anesthetist; and in a third hospital, the bottleneck was the room itself.

- In the ED of a hospital, the bottleneck was the emergency physician.

- In a specialty clinic, an expensive technology (positron emission tomographic scan) was the bottleneck.

- In a highway system, an intersection is a bottleneck.

- In a supermarket, a bottleneck could be a cashier or shelf space.

- In an office of health insurance claims, the bottleneck was the lawyers who had to approve every settlement.

- In an airport, during peak times, the bottleneck is the runway.

- In a large HMO outpatient clinic, the bottleneck was physicians.

- In a hospital obstetrics-gynecology ED, the bottleneck was the imaging services; in another hospital, the bottleneck was the attending surgeon.

We can identify several situations with organizational bottlenecks:

Shortage of a Critical Resource

A resource constraint (a bottleneck or internal constraint) could be a specific employee, a group of employees, or equipment shortage that makes it a system constraint: for example, a highly skilled surgeon in a hospital, a magnetic resonance imager in a hospital, the cleaning crew of the ORs, the operators of a pit stop in a car race, or a modem in a communication network. It is difficult to open a bottleneck simply by adding resources because it may require extensive capital or long training periods if the bottleneck is a highly skilled professional.

Permanent Bottlenecks

In the following situations, a permanent resource constraint and a *permanent bottleneck* exist:

- An *expensive resource* is always in a state of a permanent bottleneck. Some physicians have rare and unique expertise and knowledge. They quickly become internal bottlenecks because of the demand targeted at them. Likewise the situation for senior partners in law firms or accounting firms.

- *Anesthetists* are a permanent bottleneck in many practices because of their short supply.

- *Sales and marketing personnel* are bottlenecks in their systems. The potential demand for salespeople derives from leads reaching their desks from potential customers, from meetings in trade shows, and from customer lists. The effective demand is virtually infinite relative to the available sales force, and as such they are permanent bottlenecks (Pass and Ronen, 2003).

- *Research and development personnel* face an excessive demand for their abilities, talent, and services. The demand stems from customer orders, from ideas of research and development personnel themselves, from ideas of the sales force, and from continual requests for changes and improvements. This turns them into permanent bottlenecks.

- The *dentists* are frequently the permanent bottleneck in a dental practice.

Peak Time Resource Constraints

As opposed to a situation where there is a constant shortage of a critical resource over time, resource constraints during peak time are characterized by shortages in specified times. During the other times, the critical resources are not system bottlenecks (Ronen, Coman, and Schragenheim, 2001). This situation arises, for example, in a hospital ED during an accident with many victims, the tables in a restaurant at peak times, employees in a tax preparation firm during tax season, and the like. In these work environments, there are resources that are at excess capacity most of the time and at shortage during peak times. System managers must exercise two types of policies: one for times of excess capacity, and the other for peak demand. Good management of such situations requires, among other things, differential pricing of goods and services according to different demand periods. The issue of peak time management is detailed in Chapter 6.

Seasonality

Some examples of peak time management relate to seasonality where different seasons exhibit different demand patterns. This is a special case of peak time management. During the winter season, for example, there is a peak caused by the flu incidence, requiring special arrangements at hospital EDs and internal medicine wards, as well as enough flu vaccines and medications.

Discrete Events of Resource Constraints

Even firms with excess capacities occasionally face a shortage of a critical resource due to unforeseen circumstances such as natural disasters, a breakdown of equipment, or labor disputes.

The above situations demonstrate the need to develop a decision-making method for an environment with resource constraints, whether continuous or temporary.

We should point out that a constraint must be clearly defined. A shortage of highly skilled personnel does not define a constraint of an OR. The definition must be more specific. For example, we should specify if the bottleneck is the surgeons, the anesthetist, the nurses, surgical kits, or the room itself. A *control test to identify the constraint* is a test of "more or less." We must answer the question: If we could increase the capacity of the resource identified as the bottleneck, would the throughput of the whole system increase? If we reduce the capacity of this resource, will the system throughput decrease? If the answer is yes, this resource is indeed a system bottleneck.

Market Constraint

A market constraint is a situation of an excess capacity of production or of providing a service in which the supply exceeds the demand. This raises the need to increase demand. Another related situation is one where the unavailability of materials or components constrains the system. This is also a case of a market constraint where the market is that of the materials or components.

Market constraint: A situation where the market demand is less than the output capacity of each resource. Thus, market demand is the constraint that prevents the system from achieving its goal.

Let us examine the example of Figure 4.2 and change the market demand from 300 patients to 25, as depicted in Figure 4.3. The market constrains the system and prevents it from achieving its goal. Each one of the three resources has an excess capacity. This situation is referred to as a "market constraint," "excess capacity," or "external constraint." To validate that we have correctly identified the market as the system constraint, we must apply the *control test*: If market demand would increase, can we increase the system

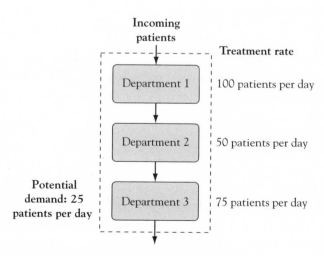

Figure 4.3. A System with a Market Constraint.

throughput? If the answer is yes (which it is in this case), then indeed the market is the system constraint.

Most industrial and service organizations today face a situation where the market is the constraint, mainly because of global competition. Only a fraction of organizations can afford to be in a situation where an internal constraint will force it to turn away demand because of lack of resources. This will be further discussed in Chapter 18. In the health care industry, we face both resource and market constraints. In a hospital, for example, the OR may be a bottleneck whereas the internal medicine wards are at excess capacity (market constraint). At the same time, the hospital laboratory may have a market constraint after 3 P.M. because of low demand for tests.

Policy Constraint

A policy constraint prevents the system from achieving its goal. The inappropriate policy is a system constraint. Every organization should set policy in important areas. A policy that may have been appropriate in previous years may become a policy constraint when changes occur in the business environment. In other situations, a local view may cause policy constraints that drive the system toward suboptimization.

Policy constraint: Adopting an inappropriate policy that limits system performance and achievement of goals and that may push in a direction that is against the organizational goal. This is also known as *policy failure*.

A hospital is reimbursed according to length of stay. This policy leads to a lack of motivation to discharge patients early, which in turn leads to longer hospital stays that increase the incidence of hospital-acquired infections. This is obviously working against the hospital's goal, which is to provide the best medical care to a maximum number of patients.

A hospital director in an effort to contain costs decides to forbid any overtime work for *all* hospital staff (bottlenecks and non-bottlenecks alike). This constrains the number of patients who could be operated on daily, increases their waiting time for surgery, causes some of them to go to another hospital, and results in adverse effects for some patients. This decision is obviously a policy constraint that works against the hospital's goals.

The purchasing department of a large HMO instructs its staff not to process any purchase orders between the 25th and the end of the month. Such a policy is intended to improve cash flow and may be a reasonable one when purchasing major and important items (type A in a Pareto analysis). However, with inexpensive items like office supplies and the like, delays resulting from this policy constraint may harm the organization because it may delay providing appropriate services to the patient population.

Here are more examples of policy constraints:

• Premiums and norms that depend only on the quantity processed are a policy constraint. They can lead to a drive to increase throughput without considering quality and create an incentive to create outputs for which there is no demand.

• Setting standards that each employee must achieve may lead to "pegging," meaning that where there is no incentive to exceed the standard, employees will be satisfied when they have reached the standard.

• Continuing to invest in a failing project just because large amounts have already been invested in it (the "sunk-cost" effect) is a policy failure.

• Across-the-board personnel cuts of 10 percent are a policy constraint that may be counterproductive for the organization.

Any policy that is applied across the board throughout an organization is suspected of being a policy constraint. What is right for one department may not be right for another. Differential management is needed. A common policy constraint is the use of local performance measures or measures that are not congruent with the organizational goal (see Chapter 13). Measuring people, units, or processes with inappropriate measures leads to wrong decisions and is a detriment to achieving goals.

To ascertain that we have correctly identified a policy constraint as a system constraint, we apply a *control test*: If we could "break" the policy constraint, could we *increase throughput* and improve the firms' value? If the answer is yes, then there is a policy constraint that is a system constraint.

Dummy Constraint

A dummy constraint exists where system throughput is constrained because of a resource whose cost is marginal.

Dummy constraint: A situation where the system bottleneck is a relatively cheap resource compared with other resources in the system.

A hospital OR used for coronary angiographies was not managing to keep its schedule of procedures. A careful analysis showed that all the needed resources—surgeons, radiologists, nurses, surgical kits, and the like—were available. Even though the OR staff was available, there were times that the OR was not being used. It turned out that the unused time resulted from waiting for a cleaning person to clean the OR between procedures. The problem arose from the desire of management to reduce cleaning costs. Initially there were two cleaners during every shift: one was in the OR and the other in the intensive care rooms. A work-flow analysis showed that labor utilization of each cleaner was only 40 percent. This was disturbing to management, and they laid off one cleaner, leaving the second responsible for both the OR and the intensive care rooms. When cleaning was needed in the OR, the cleaner was occasionally busy in the intensive care rooms, and vice versa. An inexpensive resource, the cleaning person, became a system constraint, resulting in reduced OR productivity and throughput.

In a hospital internal medicine ward, blood specimens were placed in special trays to be transported to the lab. A shortage of trays caused delays in collecting the blood specimens from patients, causing delays in receiving results, which in turn caused delays in providing treatment or discharging patients. An inexpensive resource, trays, prevented the ward from operating efficiently.

An ED had a shortage of clerical personnel for discharging patients (to the wards or home) that resulted in delays of patient discharges and overcrowding of the department. A clerk is a relatively inexpensive resource compared with physicians and nurses.

A shortage in phone lines, fax machines, copying paper, printers, digital thermometers, blood pressure monitors, and the like are all dummy constraints. These are relatively cheap resources compared with the costs of other resources and compared with the potential effect of decreased throughput.

To determine that a dummy constraint is indeed a system constraint, we must apply the control test: If we could break the dummy constraint, could we increase throughput and enhance company value? If the answer is yes, then the dummy constraint is indeed a system constraint.

Tools for Identifying Constraints in the Health Care System

A constraint can be identified in several ways:

• *Ask the field people*. The workers in the field know the work, and using their experience and intuition will usually pinpoint the real bottleneck.

- *Tour the work area.* Touring the work area helps identify the bottleneck. This is usually the place where patients, materials, or paperwork pile up.

- *Ask the evening cleaning crew.* They usually know where the inventory or paperwork is piled up.

Several methodological ways of identifying constraints are described below:

- Process flow diagram

- Time analysis

- Load analysis

- Cost-utilization (CUT) diagram

Process Flow Diagram

A process flow diagram is a basic flowchart to describe the work flow in a system (see Figure 4.4). It depicts the stages of the process and the decision nodes. To facilitate identifying a bottleneck, it is recommended to simplify the process flow diagram (eight to twelve steps) to reflect only the *main work process* and ignore marginal ones and "unusual" ones.

It is recommended that each work step include the following two time measurements:

1. Actual processing time of step (net time)

2. Total time that includes the actual processing time and the waiting time (gross time)

The basic process flow diagram can be expanded into a two-dimensional diagram that presents the various units in the organization that perform the various tasks (see Figure 4.5). It has an added importance in improving communication within the organization and is a simple visual aid that helps people understand the work flow. The actual drawing of a process flow diagram in itself provides people with

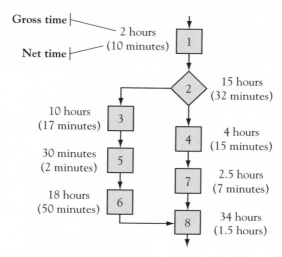

Figure 4.4. A Process Flow Diagram.

new insights about their work process, which has been a routine for them for many years. It can even happen that during the initial drawing of a process flow diagram, one can identify the system bottleneck.

Time Analysis

Analyzing the gross time of a typical entity (patient, record, product, customer, batch, and so forth) in different parts of the system enables identification of the station where it spent the longest time. This station could be a system constraint. The long time is usually due to waiting in line before the constraint. For example, step 8 in Figure 4.5 has the longest (gross) duration of 34 hours and is thus suspected to be a system constraint.

Load Analysis

Load analysis (capacity utilization) is a simple and clear tool for identifying the system bottleneck that is the most heavily used resource in the system. To determine the load on resources in the system during the time of analysis, several data must be examined:

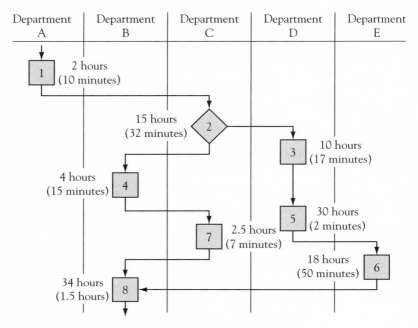

Figure 4.5. A Two-Dimensional Process Flow Diagram.

- Total number of labor hours during the time period analyzed

- The overall planned work: number of units we plan to work on (provide service, produce, plan, and so forth) with a specification of quantities by type of customer, product, development task, or other service

- A table describing the effort in labor hours that each resource is required to invest in each product, customer, development, and the like

A manufacturer of surgical equipment receives many orders for surgical kits, and the question is whether they can produce the entire order. The manufacturer has 190 monthly labor hours at its disposal. The orders for the following month consist of 100 kits of type A, 50 of type B, 25 of type C, and 200 of type D. The company has four production stations. Table 4.1 provides the number of labor hours required for the assembly of each kit type at each station.

In the load analysis table in Table 4.2, we multiply, for each kit and each resource, the planned quantity by the labor hours of the resource for the kit. As a second step, we add all the labor hours invested by the resource in the different kits and divide by the total number of labor hours per month: 190. The load analysis shows that station 3 cannot perform all its tasks to meet market demand. It is the most heavily utilized station and is therefore the system constraint.

Using a Cost-Utilization Diagram to Identify the Constraint

A cost-utilization (CUT) diagram of a system is a simple graphic tool first developed for analyzing computer systems of an organization (Borovitz and Ein-Dor, 1977) and later adapted for analysis of system constraints (Ronen and Spector, 1992). A CUT diagram is a bar graph (histogram) where every bar represents a resource. The height of the bar represents the resource utilization (load) between 0 and 100 percent. The width of each bar represents the relative cost of the resource. The relative costs of the resources can be defined in several ways:

• Based on the marginal cost of each resource: the cost associated with adding one unit of the resource. This could be adding one

Table 4.1. Labor Hours per Unit per Station.

| Surgical Kit | Labor Hours per Surgical Kit | | | |
	Station 1	Station 2	Station 3	Station 4
A	0.60	0.15	0.73	—
B	0.35	0.72	1.18	0.50
C	1.60	—	1.36	2.56
D	0.20	0.06	0.44	0.41

Table 4.2. Load Analysis

Surgical Kit	Quantity	Station 1	Station 2	Station 3	Station 4
A	100	100 × 0.60 = 60	100 × 0.15 = 15	100 × 0.73 = 73	—
B	50	50 × 0.35 = 17	50 × 0.72 = 36	50 × 1.18 = 59	50 × 0.50 = 25
C	25	25 × 1.60 = 40	—	25 × 1.36 = 34	25 × 2.56 = 64
D	200	200 × 0.20 = 40	200 × 0.06 = 12	200 × 0.44 = 88	200 × 0.41 = 82
Total hours		157	63	254	171
Load (%)		83	33	134	90

employee to a workstation or adding a machine or component. This is the recommended approach for using a CUT diagram.

- Based on the total cost of each resource.
- Based on the amortization of each resource.
- Based on a cost ratio derived from subjective assessments of the people preparing the diagram. This represents the subjective view of the relative cost or relative scarcity of the resource.

Note that the order of bars on the horizontal axis is of no importance. In a sequential process, we can arrange the bars according to the sequence of resources in the process. To understand the value of the CUT diagram, let us examine the process depicted in Figure 4.6. Let us consider the load and resource cost of the various departments (see Table 4.3). The CUT diagram of Figure 4.7 is based on the above data. It shows that the bottleneck is department E and that there are no capacity problems in the other four departments.

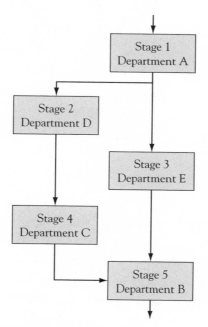

Figure 4.6. A System and Its Work Process.

Table 4.3. Load Analysis with a Bottleneck.

Resource	Load (%)	Cost of Resource ($ thousands)
Department A	55	100
Department B	80	50
Department C	45	40
Department D	65	100
Department E	100	280

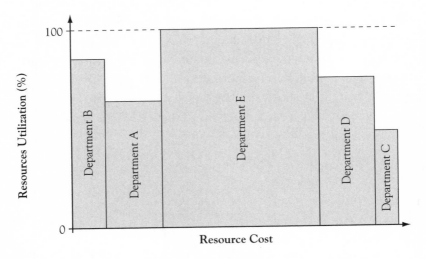

Figure 4.7. CUT Diagram of a System with a Resource Constraint.

Figure 4.7 depicts a situation where the expensive bottleneck is the only resource at full use. Such situations arise in ORs where the surgeon or the anesthetist is a bottleneck whereas other resources are only partially utilized, in an airline where all the planes are fully utilized and the crews only partially, or in an imaging department where one piece of equipment is fully utilized and others are not. In such a situation, the following points need attention:

- Management must decide if the organizational constraint should be an internal resource constraint or whether strategically and economically it should operate at excess capacity.
- When a system has excess capacity in non-bottleneck components, management should consider selling or renting out this excess capacity in an external market. For example, if a surgeon is the bottleneck in the OR of a hospital and as a result the OR is underutilized, it may be worthwhile to rent out the OR time to external surgeons. Alternatively, an effort could be made to elevate this constraint by hiring an additional surgeon.
- One must evaluate the selling price of services or products that use the bottleneck resources.

Let us examine another system whose process is also represented in Figure 4.6. However, the load relations of the resources and their relative prices are different. Table 4.4 presents the new data. The CUT diagram for Table 4.4 is presented in Figure 4.8. The CUT diagram shows that the system has market demands that are lower than the capacity of each of its resources. The system has a market constraint and is at excess capacity. The throughput is 80 percent of the potential throughput of the component with the highest use.

The following points deserve attention:

- The organization must decide whether the constraint should be external (market) while considering the excess capacity.

Table 4.4. Load Analysis in a System with a Market Constraint.

Resource	Load (%)	Cost of Resource ($ thousands)
Department A	65	10
Department B	80	17
Department C	45	15
Department D	70	15
Department E	55	28

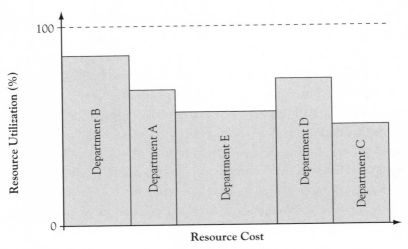

Figure 4.8. CUT Diagram of a System with a Market Constraint.

• Management must analyze whether the market constraint is temporary or permanent and identify the reasons for its existence (internal sources such as quality, price, or response time or external factors like competitors, demographic or regulatory changes, or change in customer tastes and preferences).

• Management should consider the option of taking on additional work while making sure this does not create a bottleneck. The planning phase requires reserving the capacity to protect the process throughput from fluctuations (see Chapter 14).

Let us now consider a third example whose process is also described in Figure 4.6. The load and cost figures are different from the previous examples, as shown in Table 4.5. The CUT diagram presented in Figure 4.9 illustrates the system's problem. System output is constrained by an inexpensive resource. Only a small investment may be needed to increase capacity in department E, leading to increased system output. This is a dummy constraint.

Here are some uses of the CUT diagram for two decision problems.

Table 4.5. Load Analysis for a System with a Dummy Constraint.

Resource	Load (%)	Cost of Resource ($ thousands)
Department A	65	200
Department B	75	350
Department C	40	380
Department D	70	590
Department E	100	10

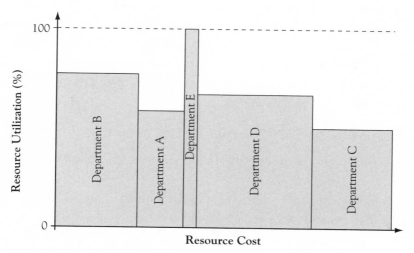

Figure 4.9. CUT Diagram of a System with a Dummy Constraint.

Investment Decisions

The CUT diagram serves as a tool for investment decisions that relate to one or more components of the process. We should assure that the additional throughput achieved by breaking the constraint is worth the investment. Frequently if we, for example, double the resource of the bottleneck, we do not double the system throughput because the bottleneck may have shifted to another resource or step, and the gains in throughput are only marginal. Following the investment, we have to analyze the effects of the new capacity on the entire system. This model will assist decision makers in deciding whether to also invest in another department that may now become the new bottleneck.

Make-or-Buy Decisions

This tool is also useful in assessing the impact of a decision to provide a new service or produce a new product on the overall loads of the system. The new load will form the basis for a make-or-buy decision. This tool is also useful for choosing the products or services to be delegated to subcontactors.

The CUT diagram also assists in making a decision on stopping a service or production of a certain product and strategic decisions on price policy and its effects on operational loads (see details in Chapter 16).

Routine Use of CUT Diagrams

CUT diagrams can be employed routinely using the following steps:

1. Construct a table that compiles the various resources, the load percentage of each, and their cost.

2. Draw a histogram where every resource has a bar whose height represents load and width represents cost. Draw the 100 percent load line.

3. Identify any problems that emerge in the diagram (dummy constraints, large excess capacity, and so forth).

4. Decide how to rectify the problem.

Chapter Summary

Management by constraints is a management theory that focuses on a system's constraints, which are the factors that limit and constrain system performance. Constraints can be categorized into four types: resource constraints (bottlenecks), market constraints (excess capacity), policy constraints, and dummy constraints.

The most common constraints in the competitive business environment are market constraints. However, there are many instances where resource constraints and bottlenecks are the causes that prevent the system from achieving its goal. There are always bottlenecks in the areas of research and development and sales and marketing. Expensive resources or temporary loads during peak times bring resource constraints on the system. Dummy constraints are inexpensive bottlenecks and must be quickly eliminated. Policy constraints result from policy and rules set by the organization (usually in the past) that hinder performance.

Bottlenecks can be identified by visiting the workstations and interviewing people or by using process flow diagrams, load analysis, and CUT diagrams.

5

Management by Constraints in a Bottleneck Environment

Objectives

- How to manage bottlenecks

- How to exploit constraints using Pareto analysis and strategic gating

- Why it is difficult to subordinate the system to the constraint

- How to appreciate the value of the offloading mechanism

This chapter focuses on situations where system throughput is limited because of a resource constraint (bottleneck). In these situations, one must focus on the constraining resource and manage it efficiently and effectively. Any improvement that adds effective capacity to the constraint will increase throughput to the whole organization. We begin by continuing the discussion of the steps for managing constraints listed in Chapter 4.

Step 4: Decide How to Exploit and Utilize the Constraint; "Break" Policy and Dummy Constraints

In a situation of resource shortage (human or material), the inclination is to solve the shortage by seeking additional personnel for service, sales, development, or production or by acquiring additional equipment.

The step of exploiting and utilizing the constraint means that *much more* can be done with existing resources, that is, extract significant additional output by focused management of the bottleneck resources. The decision on whether to increase resources should be postponed until after the improvement potential of the current bottleneck is fully exploited.

Improvement through exploitation can be achieved relatively fast and is, therefore, the most realistic improvement for the short term. Experience has shown that in *every* system it is possible to extract more by better system management and by focusing on existing constraints. Exploitation is performed on two dimensions: efficiency and effectiveness (see Figure 5.1). In parallel, we must break policy and dummy constraints.

- *Efficiency*: Increasing bottleneck utilization to as close as possible to 100 percent

- *Effectiveness*: Because the bottleneck cannot supply the entire demand, one must decide on the product or service mix of the bottleneck

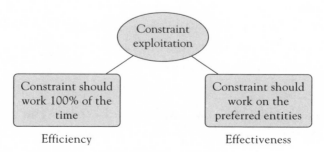

Figure 5.1. Exploiting and Utilizing the Resource.

Efficiency: Increasing Constraint Utilization

The bottleneck determines system throughput. Thus, we must make sure that it operates to the maximal possible utilization as close as possible to 100 percent of its time. The constraint is the "goose that lays golden eggs" (or the "money-printing machine") for the organization. An hour of bottleneck utilization is an hour of work for the entire system. An hour lost in the bottleneck is an hour lost for the entire system (Goldratt and Cox, 1992).

Experience gained in hundreds of organizations shows that we can significantly increase *bottleneck throughput* in sales, marketing, development, and operations *without adding resources* by better focused management of the resources (Mabin and Balderstone, 2000). For the bottleneck to work more efficiently, one can operate in two modes:

1. Increase bottleneck capacity utilization to as close as possible to 100 percent.
2. Reduce bottleneck ineffective ("garbage") time.

Increasing Bottleneck Utilization

Bottleneck utilization will be increased by measuring its idle times and analyzing these times using the Pareto focusing method.

In a large hospital, a bottleneck in patient processing was an expensive magnetic resonance imaging (MRI) machine. Measurement of its idle time revealed that the machine is idle 32 percent of the time. Idle times were handled as follows:

• *Problem classification*: Pareto classification of problems revealed that 20 percent of problems (type A problems) account for 80 percent of idle time. These problems are

1. Allocating blocks of time to wards that do not utilize their time

2. Concurrent lunch breaks of several technicians

3. Maintenance problems

• *Differential policy*: Management decided to focus only on type A problems. Other sources of idle time will be occasionally monitored to verify that they do not cause more idle time than in the past.

• *Allocation of improvement resources*: Most resources will be devoted to type A problems.

Using existing management resources, management took the following steps:

1. MRI blocks were eliminated, and imaging was scheduled by appointment or by emergent cases.

2. Lunch breaks were staggered across three hours so that the bottleneck could operate at full capacity during lunch time.

3. Maintenance problems were monitored, and preventive maintenance was undertaken.

4. The maintenance department was instructed to give the MRI top priority.

The operating rooms (ORs) in a public hospital were a bottleneck and were idle 42 percent of the time. The main causes of the idle times were the wait for the cleaning crew (dummy constraint) and cancelled operations by the anesthetist who discovered that the patients did not undergo all prerequired tests (that is, they arrived with "incomplete kits," see Chapter 12). Idle time of the ORs drastically decreased when another cleaning crew was designated for the OR area, and a preoperative clinic made sure that a "complete kit" was created about one week before the scheduled surgery.

Reducing Ineffective ("Garbage") Time

The "garbage plant" is similarly defined, including the wasted materials and all other expenses. Ineffective time may vary in different ways.

Garbage time: When the bottleneck is devoted to activities that do not add value to the customer, the service, or the product or to activities it should not perform. This is the ineffective time of the bottleneck.

In a group dental practice, the dentists were frequently occupied with typing reports and scheduling patient appointments, which mostly can be done by a secretary.

The bottleneck in the office of Minnesota State Claims was the attorneys who had to sign off on every claim. This created a big backlog and delays in claim processing. Once authority was delegated to claims specialists, claims were processed much faster.

The sales personnel of a large multinational pharmaceutical firm estimated that 50 percent of their time was ineffective. This was similar to assessments in other similar firms. They applied the focusing method as follows:

Classifying Garbage Time Causes

The various causes were classified into A, B, and C groups. Group A consisted of 20 percent of causes, accounted for 80 percent of the garbage time, and included the following:

- Working with an incomplete kit. The sales force approached customers without acquiring all the knowledge and information on their needs, thus requiring frequent repeated visits. The information was occasionally available in the firm but did not reach the sales department.

- Inappropriate identification of the decision maker in customers' organizations
- Dealing with administrative and logistic problems of the customer (shipments, missing items, inquiries, and so forth)

Differential Policy

The firm decided to treat only the above three causes of garbage time.

Resource Allocation

A majority of management resources was devoted to decreasing the above three problems.

As a result of applying the focusing method, the garbage time of the sales force was reduced from 50 percent to 40 percent, which is equivalent to increasing the sales force by 20 percent. The volume of contribution to profit increased as a result.

In a large hospital, the major tasks of the chief nurse are to manage the facility and mentor the junior nurses. It turns out that 30 percent of her time is wasted on dealing with paperwork of newly admitted patients. This paperwork can be easily handled by one of the regular veteran nurses.

In the surgical department of a hospital, the bottleneck was the anesthetist. About 30 percent of his time was considered ineffective: 10 percent because of a lack of synchronization with other OR staff (surgeons, nurses), 10 percent because of incomplete kits, and 10 percent was wasted between the end of one surgery and the beginning of the next one (suturing to cutting).

Effectiveness

Because the bottleneck cannot supply the entire demand, one must decide on the product or service mix or the projects or customers on whom the bottleneck will operate.

Strategic gating: A process of prioritization that defines the value of the different tasks, products, services, projects, or customers that are valuable to the organization and decides *which will be carried out* and in which priority and the ones that will not be carried out.

In a large firm that produces medical devices, the research and development department was working simultaneously on four innovative products, each being a potential breakthrough in its area. Estimating the load in the development department indicated that the timetables dictated by the market would allow the development of only two products. A strategic gating decision was to halt the development of two of the four products. This decision eventually resulted in a competitive time to market of one of the devices, enhancing the value of the firm.

A health maintenance organization (HMO) was planning a campaign to increase membership. They listed seventy-five big firms and twenty smaller ones as potential targets for marketing. They had only a small window of time in which workers in these firms were allowed to change carriers. The short time frame and the large number of potential organizations made it necessary for them to prioritize the firms by size and ease of attracting their workers. Using an "easy-important" table (see Chapter 3), they focused on thirty large firms and ten small ones where they applied aggressive marketing while totally ignoring the other firms. This strategic gating resulted in an astonishing 65 percent recruiting rate.

In a large downtown supermarket, there are 15,000 stock-keeping units. The bottleneck of the supermarket is shelf space. The purchaser for this supermarket is swamped with suppliers knocking on her door, representing 150,000 relevant stock-keeping units. They needed strategic prioritization to choose products that will most contribute to increased profit. Every product has a potential contribution, but a shortage of shelf space required prioritization that excludes some products altogether.

Prioritization Methods: Strategic Gating

There are several methods for prioritization. We discuss a few.

- *Use the Pareto diagram.* A Pareto diagram can be drawn for the potential contribution to the system or for any other relevant measure. This is a simple and fast method, but it does not take into account the bottleneck time needed for each activity.
- *Use a focusing table (easy-important) and a focusing matrix.* The potential tasks or projects are listed in a focusing table. For every task, we list the importance (expected contribution volume, value-enhancing capability, or contribution to achieving company goals) on a scale of 1 to 5. Then we list the ease of achieving each task (use of bottleneck time) on a scale of 1 to 5. The various tasks are mapped on a focusing matrix that helps prioritize the preferred tasks.

It is preferred to measure importance and ease of implementation on objective dimensions: value enhancement or contributions. Ease of implementation can be measured, for example, by work hours needed by the bottleneck resource.

The information technology (IT) department of a large private hospital was the bottleneck for many activities. Every department and every ward wanted the development of numerous IT applications. Management had to prioritize projects for development. The ease of development was assessed by the number of person-hours of the development bottlenecks, and the importance was assessed by the contribution to hospital profits in the next three years of implementing these applications. As a result of this prioritization, out of 1,500 projects and applications that have been waiting for months in the IT department, 750 were chosen, and the waiting time decreased dramatically.

• *Use specific contribution.* The tool for ranking the most valuable products, jobs, and customers is their specific contribution.

The *specific contribution* (the contribution per unit of resource) of a product, tasks, service, or customer is the expected contribution divided by the time investment of the resource.

$$\text{Specific contribution} = \frac{\text{contribution}}{\text{time invested by bottleneck}}$$

In a strategic gating process, we calculate the specific contribution for every product, service, task, or customer. We then choose the combination of items with the highest specific contribution until constraint capacity is reached. The specific contribution can assist the sales department in deciding on which customers to focus the scarce sales resources. The marketing and development departments can use the specific contribution in new product development decisions.

Note that the use of "specific contribution" is the correct and complete process for prioritization (Geri and Ronen, 2005). Using a focusing table is a good approximation when it is difficult to quantify performance measures. In a situation where the focusing table and focusing matrix are constructed by performance measures such as contribution on the one hand and work hours on the other, the graphic representation is an important step toward calculating the specific contribution. Many organizations prefer to perform strategic gating at the level of a focusing table and focusing matrix because the graphic representation makes it easier to decide.

The research and development department of an electronics firm that specializes in imaging technology was considering four projects, which are presented in Table 5.1. Prioritization, determined by the specific contribution, will be as follows:

1. MRI 1

2. MRI 2

3. CT scan 1

4. CT scan 2

In large supermarkets, shelf space is the resource constraint. Product prioritization should consider specific contribution per shelf length in order to maximize overall contribution to profits.

A private hospital specializes in providing surgical services where external surgeons bring in external patients. The ORs are the system bottleneck. For several years, it was believed that gynecological surgical procedures were the most profitable for the hospital. A specific contribution analysis was performed, and operations were ranked by descending order of specific contribution per hour of OR in a Pareto diagram (presented in Figure 5.2). As can be seen, the high-

Table 5.1. Imaging Projects.

Project	Contribution ($ thousands)	Development Effort (person-years)	Specific Contribution ($ thousands per person-year)
CT scan 1	56	0.5	112.0
MRI 1	2,470	1.0	2,470.0
CT scan 2	345	5.0	69.0
MRI 2	1,250	2.0	612.5

est specific contribution is from vascular surgery, then neurosurgery; orthopedics; ear, nose, and throat; and urology. Gynecology is only in sixth place. This graph can easily help the hospital prioritize the types of operations they want to focus on. Within eighteen months, OR use increased by 17 percent, and hospital profits have almost tripled!

The Mirabilis Effect

Any strategic gating decision can be a difficult one for decision makers. A decision on *what to produce and what to focus on* always carries with it the complementary decision of *what to give up*. Because the gating decision is done under conditions of uncertainty, there is always the doubt of correctly assessing the expected contributions and effort needed. There is always the fear that the product

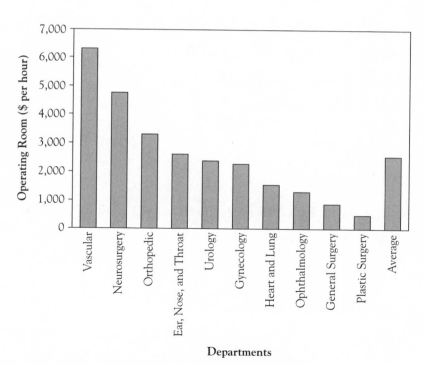

Figure 5.2. A Pareto Diagram of Specific Contribution.

rejected through prioritization could have been Mirabilis. (Mirabilis was a small Israeli high-tech firm that developed the ICQ software and was sold to AOL for over $400 million). However, if this were the case, this product should have been assessed a higher expected contribution, resulting in a higher specific contribution. The fact that a product is not assessed a higher value indicates the presence of other products that seem to have a higher success probability during the time of decision.

Firms need managerial maturity to realize that physical rules cannot be bent, and there is no system that can perform all the tasks that one would want. If management will not engage in prioritization, this will happen on its own in the field without regard to global considerations for the benefit of the organization. In cases of indecision, the development of services or products will be delayed or the focus will not be on the right customers.

The Global Decision-Making Method

The specific contribution is only one part of tactical and strategic prioritization and screening of tasks, services, or products. As we shall see in Chapter 16, the global decision-making process includes three steps: making a global economic decision from the CEO's perspective; making strategic considerations; and if needed, changing local performance measures.

Make a Global Economic Decision from the CEO's Perspective

In this process, we evaluate the decision from a global perspective by looking at the whole system. The process may use specific contributions.

Make Strategic Considerations

We must consider long-term and other strategic considerations, only after we can assess the financial implications of priority changes in the decision of the previous step.

When one or more of the alternatives in the prioritization process has indirect marketing implications or broader strategic implications, we must expand the analysis of their expected contributions and prepare a "mini-business plan" for each alternative.

Change, If Needed, Local Performance Measures

Local performance measures may occasionally prevent correct prioritization. For example, prioritizing customers by a local performance measure of sales volume requires a change to prioritizing them according to their specific contribution.

Breaking Policy and Dummy Constraints

Bottlenecks must be exploited efficiently and effectively. Dummy and policy constraints must be broken. The dummy constraint of the cleaning person in the OR in the example given in Chapter 4 can be immediately remedied by hiring additional personnel. One does not need an economist to perform a cost-benefit analysis to justify this solution.

Policy constraints are a bit more difficult to deal with. For example, overtime work (which is usually needed at the end of quarters or the end of a year) can be eliminated by a policy that differentiates between work centers that are bottlenecks and other work centers. This allows the manager to manage a "petty cash" account of the overtime budget for the bottlenecks.

Step 5: Subordinate the System to the Constraint

Once we focus on the constraint (bottleneck) and improve its management, we need to create a policy for managing and operating noncritical resources. The remaining resources should *serve and assist the bottleneck.* In a group dental practice, the dentists are the system constraints, so the other workers (hygienists, assistants, secretary) should all assist the dentists.

The noncritical resources must be available to assist system constraints, especially at peak times. For example, in peak tourist seasons, the runways of an airport are the bottleneck. All other workers and managers must contribute their share to efficiently exploit the runway times for fast and safe takeoffs and landings.

> Henry Ford offered customers the Model T Ford "in any color the customer wants, as long as it is black. " Henry Ford's policy resulted from subordination to the assembly-line constraint that could not keep up with market demand. This was a resource constraint. To maximize throughput, it was important for Ford not to change models during production. This policy assured achieving the goal of maximizing the profit and value for the Ford Motor Company by subordinating the whole system to production.
>
> Henry Ford's failure was that he stuck to his policy even when new competitors entered the market, and the constraint became a market constraint. This resulted in a steep drop in sales and market share. The right step would have been to realize that there was now a market constraint and to subordinate the system to this constraint. Ford should have switched to producing a variety of cars that were demanded by customers and were offered by his competitors: different styles, colors, or amenities.
>
> In the development of a new drug, a pharmaceutical firm should be driven by the market rather than by innovation for the sake of innovation and prestige.
>
> In an OR in a hospital, the bottleneck could be the anesthetists, nurses, or the OR capacity itself. Management must identify the bottleneck and subordinate all others to serve and assist the bottleneck to ensure it functions efficiently.

From our experience with the previous example, implementing the subordination phase may be difficult in certain cases. If the bottleneck is the senior surgeon, we did not experience any subordination problems. However, in cases where the anesthetist was the bottleneck, it was difficult to subordinate the surgeons to the specific timetable of the anesthetist.

Additional examples:

- Imaging technicians' work shifts should be planned according to the timetables of the senior radiologist if he or she is the system bottleneck.
- In maintenance, priority should be given to the bottleneck. When the bottleneck fails, the relevant maintenance people should drop all other tasks and assist in fixing the bottleneck because it stops all system output.
- Releasing tasks for service or development should be scheduled according to the bottleneck pace.
- If efficient use of a hospital lab calls for batches of a hundred specimens at a time, then all wards and logistics should subordinate to this constraint, even if they prefer preparing larger batches.

Subordination Mechanisms

Noncritical resources can be subordinated to an organizational constraint using the following mechanisms: tactical gating and the drum-buffer-rope (DBR) mechanism.

Tactical Gating Mechanism

To help the system perform to its utmost, the constraint must work efficiently and effectively. The rest of the system is subordinated to the constraint by a mechanism of releasing tasks into the system. This is the tactical gating mechanism. Tactical gating means the controlled release of tasks (jobs) to the system. To assure efficient operation of the bottleneck, the tactical gating mechanism will employ the following policy:

- All tasks will be released for work in the *right batch size* (see Chapter 11).

- Only tasks screened by the gating process will be released for workup.

- A task that was not screened and released by the gater will not be processed. All tasks will be released only through the body or person in charge of the gating (the "gater").

- All tasks (in development, medical service, production) will enter the system with a complete kit (see Chapter 12).

- All tasks will enter according to an appropriate *scheduling mechanism*, for example, the DBR.

Drum-Buffer-Rope Mechanism

The DBR mechanism, presented in Figure 5.3, is a scheduling mechanism for entering tasks into the system (Goldratt and Cox, 1992; Schragenheim and Ronen, 1990). It is appropriate for health care systems, service industries, production, and research and development.

The explanation of the specific terms is as follows: The *drum* provides the rhythm for the flow of tasks through the system. The system constraint determines the rate at which tasks should enter the system and flow through it. In the presence of a resource constraint, the drum will be the *work rate of the bottleneck*. In the case of a market constraint, the *rate of market demand* will dictate the pace for the whole system. Thus, the rate of inserting tasks into the system will be governed by the constraint and not by noncritical resources (see Chapter 9).

The *buffer* refers to a controlled quantity of tasks that accumulate before the bottleneck to assure it is fully utilized. The buffer serves to protect the system against fluctuations that arise from malfunctions and delays in the chain feeding the bottleneck. Such fluctuations can be caused by

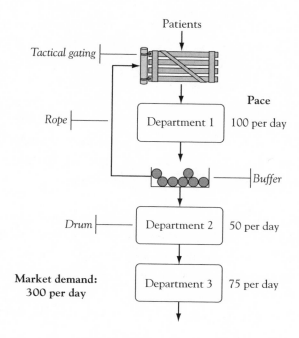

Figure 5.3. The Drum-Buffer-Rope Mechanism.

- Worker absenteeism

- Technical problem and human error in the service or production process

- Low quality of information or materials

- "No shows" of patients to the clinic or hospital

- Delays in the supply of raw materials and components

The buffer protects the bottleneck output from various fluctuations by assuring continuity of its operation. (See Chapter 14 for a discussion on fluctuations.) The size of the buffer is measured in terms of the bottleneck utilization time. To determine buffer size, we must examine the various fluctuations and time to correct them. For example, if 95 percent of fluctuations are handled within four hours, this time will determine the buffer size.

Note that there also exists an overflow buffer. In situations where there is a physical flow of materials, such as in production or logistics, malfunctions may occur in steps that come after the bottleneck. To protect for the bottleneck throughput in such situations, additional storage capacity must be arranged for the throughput of the bottleneck to provide for a continuity of work. This storage capacity is the overflow buffer.

The *rope* of the mechanism is a "logical rope" that transfers information on the situation in the buffer to the tactical gating mechanism to coordinate release of tasks into the system. When the number of tasks in the buffer becomes smaller, additional tasks are released into the system.

The following are examples of the use of the DBR mechanism:

• *In an orthodontics clinic*: The orthodontists and clerical staff of the clinic schedule patient appointments so that the orthodontists (the bottleneck) will be used and not be idle. They create a buffer of about a fifteen-minute wait for each orthodontist (about two patients waiting). If the buffer were larger, patients would complain about the excessive waiting time. In this clinic, each orthodontist (the constraint) works in three rooms in parallel. While he or she is seeing a patient in one room, the two other rooms serve as buffers where patients are waiting to be seen. In addition to the two buffer rooms, two additional patients are waiting in the waiting area. All this involves only an average of fifteen minutes' waiting time for patients but assures a high-capacity use of the orthodontists.

To reduce potential fluctuations in patient arrivals, the clinic staff call the patients the day before the scheduled appointment to verify their arrival time.

• *In an OR*: Because the duration of surgical procedures is uncertain, one should schedule patients using the DBR method.

The drum is the system bottleneck—the surgeon's rate of performing surgery. A buffer of patients (for example, on "standby") will be waiting in the preoperative room. When a patient is wheeled into the OR, the rope will signal the ward to send another patient. In cases of short operations, the buffer should be measured by time (for example, thirty minutes or a one-hour buffer). The buffer size depends on the fluctuations of the system.

• *In airports*: In airports, the runways are a bottleneck. To assure that they operate close to 100 percent capacity, arriving planes circle above the airport and serve as buffers. The buffer size will, of course, depend on safety considerations. When the buffer is full, approaching aircraft are instructed to slow down their approach, circle in wider circles, or in extreme situations, be diverted to other airports. The control tower is responsible for gating. When a plane lands, it is immediately directed to a side runway to allow for another plane to land and another plane to enter the buffer.

• *In sales*: In a multinational firm, every salesperson was in charge of forty existing customers and one hundred new potential customers. The company shifted to DBR scheduling of sales personnel. Today they operate in a focused manner where the buffer is defined by a "ten-plus-ten" approach: every salesperson is in charge of managing and preserving ten existing customers and ten potential new customers.

Step 6: Elevate and Break the Constraint

Up to this point, the previous five steps of management by constraints dealt with increasing the output of a given system, without any changes in the system itself. Now it is time for *structural changes* in the system to increase the effective capacity of the bottleneck. Increasing this capacity will increase the throughput of the whole system.

Elevating and breaking the constraint can be achieved in two ways:

- Using capital investment

- In a way that does not need investment with the use of the offloading mechanism

Elevating Using Capital Investment

An effective increase in the capacity of the constraint through the acquisition of additional resources can be achieved in one of the following ways:

- Recruiting additional staff

- Purchasing additional equipment

- Working additional shifts

- Working overtime

- Hiring subcontractors

- Outsourcing

- Recruiting distributors and value-added retailers for the sales force.

In an emergency department of a hospital, the consulting surgeons were the bottleneck. Management decided to hire some retired surgeons (who no longer operate but have great diagnostic skills) to elevate the system's constraint.

A large HMO had many litigations concerning malpractice suits. Their own attorneys became a bottleneck, so they started using the services of outside law firms.

Offloading: Delegating Mechanism Using Existing Resources

The offload process involves the transfer of work from the constraint to noncritical resources with excess capacity. From the system's perspective, it does not matter if these resources perform the task of the bottleneck at a slower pace than the bottleneck. The important fact is that they contribute to the overall output. In some cases, the offload is achieved using structured processes that need less expertise.

Offloading: Relieving the load from the bottleneck by transferring some of the workload to noncritical resources.

In many HMO clinics, physicians and nurse practitioners formed teams so that the physicians could offload some of their tasks to the nurses.

In a large HMO, a senior vice president had to sign every request for surgery in nonaffiliated hospitals. She was the bottleneck that caused delays and resulted in adverse outcomes to patients and lawsuits. She had the responsibility of verifying need, justifying surgery in a specific hospital, and determining the level of copayment. Her level of expertise was second to none, and she was indeed a scarce resource.

Offloading was achieved by training some clerks and other employees to do some of her tasks. It turned out that about 25 percent of requests were standard, and their approval process was structured and straightforward. Even though each such case required a short processing time by the specialist, offloading these cases to others released 15 percent of the specialist's time. This resulted in shorter response times to approve requests and increased system output (see Eden and Ronen, 1993).

The following are additional examples of offloading:

• A dental hygienist relieves the burden from the dentist by performing some of the dentist's tasks.

- In a supermarket during peak times, the number of registries is the bottleneck. Adding packers (baggers) at each registry offloads some of the cashiers' work to a less expensive resource.

- In university hospitals, teaching assistants and research assistants serve as offloads for the expensive resource of the professors and senior researchers who do both clinical and academic work.

- In many complex surgeries, both the beginning of the operation and the ending ("closing") are performed by junior surgeons.

Step 7: If a Constraint Is "Broken," Go Back to Step 3

If a constraint is broken, we must return to the step of identifying the new system constraint and not letting inertia become the system constraint. There is always a constraint (bottleneck) in a system. The task is to identify constraints, manage them, break them, and face a new constraint that may appear elsewhere. By moving from constraint to constraint, system output increases. Figure 5.4 describes the improvement process in the surgical department of a hospital.

In routine processes, constraints do not change frequently and are rather stable. In one-time processes (projects, sales campaigns, and the like), constraints change rapidly, and bottlenecks can move from one place to another.

Managerial inertia can be detrimental to organizational performance. An organization accustomed to a constraint being in one place may occasionally behave as if the constraint is still there, even though improvement steps broke this constraint and moved it elsewhere.

The previously mentioned example of Henry Ford exemplifies this. Even though the resource constraint at the assembly line was broken and the constraint became a market constraint, the management of the Ford Motor Company continued, out of inertia, to focus on efficient use of internal resources and did not view the market as the system constraint.

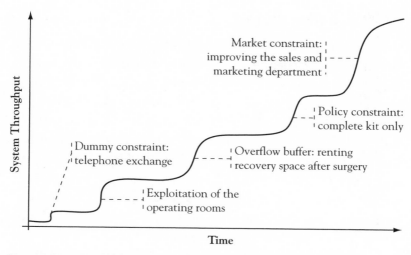

Figure 5.4. Continuous Improvement in a Surgical Department.

In an emergency department, the bottleneck was in radiology services. By using existing equipment and breaking some policy constraints, management was able to operate the two x-ray rooms in the following manner. They divided the patients needing x-ray studies into two groups: ambulatory patients and recumbent patients. The patients who could walk on their own simply walked into one designated x-ray room without assistance. The second x-ray room was devoted to recumbent patients who were wheeled into the room on specially purchased beds that did not require their transfer to a stationary bed in the room. Thus, the radiology constraint was broken.

The next constraint was a lack of expert surgical consultants. A consultant was called for consultation only when at least two or three patients required it (unless, of course, there was an emergency). The hospital assigned a special surgeon who was available in the emergency department continuously. Once the surgical consultant constraint was broken, the system faced a policy constraint in the discharge process. A team of nurses, physicians, and administrators solved the problem by redesigning the discharge process. All of these actions gradually reduced the average waiting time by 40 percent.

The "Curse of the Blessing"

Use of the techniques described in this book, such as management by constraints, frequently results in a rapid increase in throughput, a significant decrease in response times to customers, and improvement in quality. As a result of these improvements, the organization usually becomes more attractive to its customers or patients, and the demand for its services or products increases. Management that is not cautious may take on commitments beyond its new effective capacity. This may lead to delays in reaching the patients, operational difficulties, and a severe blow to the recently enhanced reputation. This is the "curse of the blessing." When the organization achieves significant improvement, it must be careful about increasing the volume of demand and always proceed gradually.

Chapter Summary

Management by constraints is the most advanced management theory today. It includes focusing steps that significantly increase system throughput within a short time by focusing on bottlenecks and other constraints. The method allows significantly improved performance of sales, marketing, service, research and development, and production systems in a relatively short time with existing resources. In the next chapter, we demonstrate how to use the theory of constraints when the market is the system constraint.

6

Management by Constraints When the Market Is the Constraint

Objectives

- Learn how to sell more using the same resources in a market-constrained environment

- Understand how to cope with peaks using the peak management approach

- Learn how solving the three questions on organizational resources can affect strategy

A system always has a bottleneck. In the previous chapter, we discussed situations involving scarce resources where the constraints were these resources. There are many situations with excess operational capacity, and then the market becomes a system constraint. Proper use of the management-by-constraints method in these situations yields improvements in throughput, quality, profits, and value of the firm.

Even private or budgeted hospitals and health maintenance organizations (HMOs) must realize that they may have excess capacity and need a strong marketing function. They should resist the temptation to lay off people during slow times. Perhaps they should consider assuming outside tasks to fill this excess capacity.

A hospital buys an expensive imaging machine. The decision is a correct one because the machine is essential for some diagnoses. However, there is not enough demand for its use. Rather than refer more patients who do not need this expensive imaging, the hospital can sell imaging services to outside sources such as HMOs and private physicians.

A technological change may cause excess capacity at bottlenecks. The development of cardiac angiography with the introduction of stents has encouraged many cardiologists to engage in this practice and to refer more patients for these techniques. As a result, cardiac surgeons who used to be a system bottleneck in the past find themselves with excess capacity because the market for their operations such as coronary bypass surgery has shrunk dramatically.

The steps of management by constraints in a system where the market is the constraint are the same as with resource constraints (Pass and Ronen, 2003):

1. Determine the system's goal.
2. Establish global performance measures.
3. Identify the system constraint.
4. Decide how to exploit the constraint; break dummy and policy constraints.
5. Subordinate the rest of the system to the constraint.
6. Elevate and break the constraint.
7. If the constraint is broken (interrupted), go back to step 3. Do not let inertia become the system constraint.

The first three steps, defining the goal and performance measures and identifying the system bottleneck, are common to both resource and market constraints. The essence of steps 4 through 6 in both situations is similar, but the methods and tools for dealing with a market constraint are different from the ones appropriate for a resource constraint. Here, too, step 4 (exploiting the constraint) can be implemented immediately. Step 5 is implemented in the intermediate term. Step 6 requires introducing more substantial changes in the system and is therefore a step aimed at the medium to long term.

Treating a market constraint is more difficult than treating a resource constraint. Managing an internal bottleneck offers management more control of what is happening in the "inner circles" of the organization, whereas some of the factors involved in dealing with a market constraint are beyond management's control.

Most non-health care organizations are faced with a market constraint. In today's fierce global competition, it is wise to have excess capacity (or protective capacity) in the production and service resources. Firms cannot usually afford a situation where the marketing and sales force managed to obtain orders while the operational factor is the constraint that prevents or delays their fulfillment.

Managing a market constraint is a key for the success of many firms and businesses, and the approaches presented in this chapter should be a valuable tool for this.

Step 4: Decide How to Exploit and Utilize the Constraint; Break Policy and Dummy Constraints

Exploiting a market constraint means exploiting the *existing* market and the *existing* sales ability more efficiently and effectively. In other words, doing more with the same resources. This exploitation will be achieved through efficient operation of marketing and sales and effective strategic marketing while eliminating policy and dummy constraints (see Figure 6.1). This implies the need to "strike" the existing market and exploit the full volume of potential contribution from existing and potential customers and products using existing personnel.

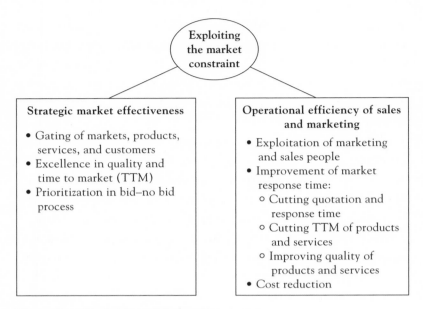

Figure 6.1. Exploiting a Market Constraint.

Marketing and Sales Efficiency

There are two elements to achieve marketing and sales efficiency. The first is exploiting marketing and sales personnel, and the second is improving response to market needs.

Exploiting Marketing and Sales Personnel

The marketing and sales personnel are usually a permanent bottleneck. As such, we must exploit them and utilize their time:

• The "garbage time" of the sales force must be reduced. Sales personnel are frequently busy with logistical problems, with time-consuming efforts to follow up on orders, and so forth. All these must be reduced.

• The sales and marketing operation should be *structured* and with stable and simple processes. In many cases, marketing and sales processes are not congruent with the organization's needs and the market. The introduction of a new service or product suffers from incomplete and disorderly marketing and from the fact that information does not reach all relevant parties. There are many examples of customers updating cashiers about various promotions.

Improving Response to Market Needs

There are many ways to improve an organization's response to market needs:

- *Reduce response times in bids, sales, and marketing.* The contribution of sales to profits can be improved by shortening response times of preparing bids, marketing, and sales processes. Despite the common claims that "every customer is different" or that "every product is unique," there is room for improving work processes so that they are uniform for every class of customers with similar features. The process of request for quotations for customers, especially in response to bids, must be structured, simple, and clear.
- *Shorten the time to market (TTM) of services and products.* A shorter TTM of new products and services enables reaching customers faster than the competition and realizing better prices. As such, operational efficiency will enhance sales. Submitting bids with fast quoted lead times for a product or service frequently makes the organization more attractive to customers and increases contribution from sales.
- *Improve service or product quality.* Improvement in the service or production processes will increase the perceived value of the firm's products or services and will increase the contribution of sales.
- *Reduce costs.* Operational efficiency by the sales and marketing personnel as well as the operational bodies can improve response times, quality, and system output.

The objective is to achieve, with existing resources and current costs, higher output, higher contributions, improved cash flow, and value enhancement for the firm. However, this is not always possible, and one must also evaluate the reduction of costs. A careful cost analysis and decisions on cost containment in the right places can significantly improve cash flow. Cost savings can sometimes permit price reduction, which may improve competitiveness. Chapter 17 discusses this further when we compare the "throughput world" with the "cost world."

Strategic Marketing Effectiveness

In the previous chapter, we introduced the concept of strategic gating, which screens and prioritizes customers or products based on their specific contribution or their positioning of the focusing matrix (easy-important). Even when an organization is at excess capacity and is facing a market constraint, the sales and marketing personnel are a permanent bottleneck. The potential demand for their services always exceeds their resources. There are always more potential customers, marketing initiatives, sales to existing customers, and offerings of new services or products than available time of sales and marketing personnel. This screening procedure is, therefore, extremely important and enables focusing on the highest specific-contribution products, services, or customers that can contribute most to increase organizational performance and value. As a result, we can state the following:

1. One should not abandon sales of services and products to customers and markets where the sales personnel are *minimally* involved, even if the *contribution volume is small*. For example, repeated sales to existing customers should not be rejected because in these sales most of the marketing and sales efforts have already been applied in the past. These are actually considered sales with a high specific contribution because of the short time invested in them by the sales or marketing people.

2. For sales of services or products or for customers who require substantial investments of time, we need to perform a prioriti-

zation process of the strategic gating. The prioritization will be carried out relative to the time that the sales and marketing personnel (the bottleneck) need to invest to achieve the contribution volume of the expected sales of these services or products.

Table 6.1 presents the calculation of the specific contribution of the various customers relative to the sales effort involved. A salesperson should first approach a customer with the highest specific contribution relative to his or her time. The top choice in Table 6.1 is HMO 2. The salesperson will then focus on HMO 1 and so forth until he or she fills up 100 percent of his or her time. This analysis must also consider strategic considerations (see the three-stage model in Chapter 16).

Strategic gating will also be performed on the variety of services and products that the organization is selling: experience shows that by focusing on a *smaller* number of services and products, it is possible to achieve a *higher* volume of contributions. Occasionally it is advisable to cease the sale of services and products whose total contribution volume is negligible. Cessation of sales can be done in two ways: one, discontinue offering them to the market, and two, if there is concern that the market will not react positively to the cessation of sales, the price of the product can be raised. If there will

Table 6.1. The Specific Contribution of Customers Relative to the Sales Effort.

Customer	Contribution to Profit ($ thousands)	Sales Effort (days)	Specific Contribution ($ per day)
HMO 1	2,345	120	19,500
HMO 2	5,600	30	186,700
Group practice	575	80	7,200
Hospital	12,650	500	2,500

be no demand at the new price, the product will fade away. However, if demand persists, then the higher price will increase contribution. This situation reveals that the previous price was too low. In many cases, raising the price does not diminish demand but rather increases it.

Note that it is common to think that stopping the sale of certain products of a product line may decrease sales of the entire line. Every situation must be examined specifically. With proper planning, it is usually possible to increase contributions.

Making Excellence in Response Times and Quality into a Strategic Leverage

Japanese firms have captured the world market in cars and home electronics through the quality of the products. Their operational excellence, which enabled them to achieve high quality while incurring low production costs, fast response times, and low inventories, established a strategic advantage in the eyes of customers who were willing to pay a premium for "made in Japan."

Superb operational ability must not rely on low costs and competitive operating expenses. The challenge is to bring the excellence in quality and operations to establish a strategic advantage for the organization.

The Mayo Clinic in Rochester, Minnesota, established a name for itself even though it is located in a remote town. It attracts patients from all over the world who are willing to pay a premium for the perceived superior quality of care.

The computer manufacturer Dell achieved fast response times and low inventory costs through efficient operations and logistics management. As a result, it captured a large market share of personal computers and servers.

The Sony Corporation was able to charge its customers a substantial premium for the perceived quality of its products in comparison with the competition.

Prioritizing in Bid–No Bid Processes

In companies where most sales are through participation in bids, there must be an important step of evaluating the intent to respond to a bid. This process is known as "bid–no bid" (or "go–no go"). The bids should be evaluated on their compatibility with the company strategy, the chances of winning, and the potential contribution to profits. Bids that do not meet the criteria should be answered with no bid, thus preventing unnecessary effort by the permanent bottlenecks of the system (marketing and sales personnel, technical experts). A policy where an organization responds positively (bids) to every request becomes a policy constraint (see also Chapter 20).

Breaking Policy and Dummy Constraints

To increase the contribution volume of sales, we must identify policy and dummy constraints that interfere with the organization's efforts to cope with the market.

- *Avoid the blind use of traditional cost accounting.* As described in Chapter 15, the blind use of classical pricing can harm an organization. There are organizations where the selling price is built on "cost-plus." The desire to *always* have the selling price above the costs (including indirect costs) may lead to erroneous decisions and loss of business opportunities.
- *Avoid giving up small customer orders.* There is no reason to reject small customers or small orders that do not take up much time of the sales and marketing bottlenecks.
- *Avoid selling only complete sets ("assortments").* Certain industries (for example, shoes and clothing) tend to sell to stores in "complete

sets" only. These sets have a predetermined assortment of styles and sizes. However, preparing a specified, nonstandard assortment according to the needs of a specific store does not take up much bottleneck time, so there is no reason not to sell what the customer wants. For example, a hospital lab may be willing to sell excess capacity to outside customers. They should not insist on selling a predetermined variety of services (tests of blood, urine, and so forth) and can afford to sell what the customers need. It is wise to follow the demand patterns so that even if a firm offers only complete sets, they should be according to actual demand.

- *Avoid selling a "complete product line or nothing."* There are companies with a policy of selling customers an entire basket of services or products or nothing at all. In many cases, selling a partial basket can yield nice profits.

- *Avoid rewarding sales personnel by sales volume.* This is one of the most common forms of incentives and rewards, but this encourages the sales force to maximize sales volume and not necessarily the total contribution to profits. There is a need to shift to a reward and measurement system where profit or contribution plays an important role.

- *Avoid rewarding sales personnel regardless of returns and cancellations.* This policy encourages salespersons to sign as many contracts as possible with many customers without checking the real need of the customers and their ability to pay. This policy constraint can be rectified by rewarding the sales force by *actual* contribution volume (subtracting returns and cancellations) and only after payment has been received.

- *Avoid dummy constraints.* For example, lack of a fax machine or other communication mode for sales personnel can be a dummy constraint.

Breaking such policy and dummy constraints as illustrated above is an important factor in increasing the volume of contribution to the organization.

Step 5: Subordinate the System to the Constraint

There is an obvious advantage for an organization that satisfies its customers' needs more than the competition. In a situation with a market constraint, the organization must *subordinate the whole system to the market,* meaning that every member of the organization must subordinate himself or herself to the market and its needs. This subordination of the organization to the market will be done in the following dimensions:

- *Customization to customer demands and needs.* In a competitive market, there is a need to customize services and products to the various needs of customers. Customization is important and especially worthwhile when the customization does not require development or marketing resources but only efforts from operational entities that are not bottlenecks. When customization requires some development, strategic gating will help decide how to best utilize the constrained development resources.
- *Fast response to customer needs.* To beat the competition, one must adjust to the due date required by the customer and subordinate the whole system to the market timetable.
- *Direct link to the end customer.* Establishing a direct link with the end customer is especially important in those cases where the organization uses external distributors to sell its services and products to end customers. The organization must then establish a permanent communications process to determine the needs of the distributors and end customers. It is worthwhile to make an effort to establish a connection with the end customers by bypassing the hurdles of the distribution channels and agents. For example, if a hospital or clinic has referrals from HMOs or other insurance companies, the hospital should establish a direct link with the insured to fully understand their needs.
- *Adjusting the organizational structure to customer types or customer needs.* To better serve the market, one must assure that the

organizational structure is compatible with customer needs. Occasionally, the organizational structure is based on a geographical segmentation or is geared toward achieving operational efficiency. It may be better to redesign the structure to reflect different customer types. For example, rather than designing a large HMO to be geographically based, where every region is assigned proportionate resources, the resource allocation should be targeted to different patient groups, such as young versus old, chronically ill versus acutely ill, men versus women.

• *Subordinating technology to market needs.* High-tech organizations have a constant conflict between the market and development departments. Many technological organizations were built on their technological know-how and development breakthrough. In such situations, development may occasionally dictate the organizational road map. Development and technology must be subordinated to the market via the marketing personnel. The services and products should be defined in harmony with marketing and development but always subordinating to the market.

• *Market segmentation and product differentiation.* In case of excess capacity, an organization can meet specific demands of different market segments by product and price differentiation. This allows the channeling of excess operational capacity toward generating additional contributions. It is essential to assure the cooperation and good will of the operations people because this segmentation causes them additional managerial complexity (see Chapter 16).

In the past, obstetrical services in a hospital had internal resource constraints, usually the obstetricians and gynecologists. The services could dictate to the customers the level of service and quality. In today's highly competitive market of hospitals, HMOs, private practices, and the like, the market has become the constraint. Hospitals have completely subordinated their operation to the market. Everything is targeted to please the potential patient: support services for the delivering mother and her family were established, hotels were built to accommodate relatives, shopping malls targeted at the baby market have been built, and so forth.

Step 6: Elevate and Break the Constraint

In this step, we need to examine how to increase the contribution from sales or services by creating added value to existing customers, introducing new products or services, approaching new markets, identifying new customers, combining marketing with new sales channels, and strategic cooperation.

This step requires establishing a *focused strategy*. Occasionally, in situations with a market constraint, organizations are tempted to "shoot in all directions," to cast a wide net and wait "until the fish are caught." Such a policy can put the bottleneck resource of sales and marketing to waste. In contrast, a focused policy targeting the main objectives and focusing the efforts on these targets usually yields better outcomes. To elevate and break the market constraint, the following steps are recommended:

1. *Establish a focused strategy*: a necessary condition for increasing profit (for details, see Chapter 18)

2. *Enter a new product or market*: mergers and acquisitions of firms that have an appropriate product or market

3. *Add marketing and sales channels*: such as a new distributor or enter the world of e-business

4. *Market segmentation and product differentiation*: every market segment has different needs and requirements; products and services must be adapted according to the targeted segments

5. *"Stretch" the brand name*: implies taking advantage of the success of one brand name to create a family of related or similar products that will be sold under the same brand name

6. *Create added value for the customer*: in this category, we can include product features that add perceived value to the customer:

Create a package of services and products that complement one another

Manage the customer's facilities, shift to outsourcing of customer activities

Manage inventory for the customer

Build customer loyalty (customer clubs)

Customer relationships management

7. *Cooperation and strategic alliances*

Step 7: If a Constraint Is Broken, Go Back to Step 3; Do Not Let Inertia Become the System Constraint

If the constraint is broken, we must look for the next constraint and manage the system accordingly. There are situations where a con-strained system loses some demand and becomes a system with excess capacity and vice versa.

Managing Marketing and Sales

Focus on most valuable customers (MVCs) as a value enhancer. Investing in marketing and sales efforts in existing customers and potential new ones enables contribution to be increased. To make the best use of the scarce time of the marketing and sales person-nel, focus on existing and potential customers with a high specific contribution. MVCs are type A customers in the Pareto analysis of the organization: about 20 percent of customers (existing and poten-tial) who contribute 80 percent of contribution volume.

> In a multinational pharmaceutical company, every salesperson han-dled forty existing customers and about a hundred potential ones.

The firm adopted a policy of focused management and shifted to a "ten-plus-ten" approach: every salesperson handles sales for ten existing customers and their retention and tries to approach ten new potential customers. The new approach resulted in an immediate increase in throughput.

Such focusing enables a better response to the needs of the MVCs:

- Establish tight personal contacts with influential people in the customer organization.

- Collect and analyze data on the customer and the relevant markets.

- Provide special service—red carpet or "VIP" treatment—to the MVCs in all units of the organization.

- Analyze MVC needs and identify channels for providing more *value to the customer.*

- Determine policy vis-à-vis the customer.

- Manage risk vis-à-vis the customer.

- Structure management of meetings with the customer.

- Structure management of contracts with the customer.

It is nearly impossible to give such VIP treatment to all customers, but it should focus on MVCs, thus enabling the contribution of sales to be increased.

Peak Management

An important area derived from management by constraints is reducing the effect of peak-time loads. Appropriate management of such systems requires differential pricing of products or services during different times. The reduction of temporary loads during peak times can be achieved using the following steps (Ronen, Coman, and Schragenheim, 2001):

- *Stretch peak times*. Stretching peak times allows work to be spread over a longer period. For example, to overcome the load on a clinic during peak hours, the clinic can move back the start time of employees in certain departments and move up the opening time of the clinic (see also Chapter 11). Another example is a private hospital where the operating room (OR) moved to a 6:00 A.M. to 11:00 P.M. schedule of performing surgery.
- *Plan capacity*. It is common to plan capacity for an average load. This results in excess capacity during slow periods and to resource constraints during peak periods. Good planning should provide for adequate service and performance at all times. Hence, a strategic decision of planning capacity to provide for peak times can reduce or even prevent the peak-time loads. Examples can be found in walk-in clinics, fast food restaurants, banks, and pharmacies. Planning should include providing the infrastructure for peak times and a mechanism for adjusting the level of the labor force to vary by load.
- *Transfer load to low-load periods*. An appropriate pricing or reward policy can divert some of the demand to low-load periods. Examples include the pricing policies of airlines and phone companies.
- *Use temporary help*. Peak times are characterized by a lack of production or service resources in certain distinct periods. Using temporary help can remedy these situations. Tax firms hire temporary help during tax season, restaurants hire temporary help during lunch breaks, and so forth.

In a work environment with obvious peak times, some resources are at excess capacity most of the time and in shortage during the peak times. As a result, management must handle two types of policy: one for times of excess capacity and one for shortage of resources. In emergency departments (EDs) of hospitals, there is a big variation in arrival times between day and night. These EDs are managed with excess capacity ("day ED") on the one hand and as an ED oper-ating under resource constraints ("night ED") on the other.

Where Should the Constraint Be Located?

An important strategic issue is where to locate the system con-straint. Until now, we considered situations with a given system, and the goal was to improve it. To strategically place the constraint, we must consider three strategic questions about the resources of the organization:

- Where should the constraint be?

- Where is the constraint now?

- How can we transfer the constraint to the proper place?

The first question—Where should the constraint be?—can be broken down into two parts: does the constraint have to be an inter-nal one (resource constraint) or an external one (market con-straint), and if the constraint is a resource constraint, which resource has to be the constraint? The advantages of placing the constraint in the system as an internal bottleneck are obvious: sav-ings in resources and control over demand and over the system. This translates into the ability to sort and screen orders, customers, services, and products and to better control the planning and imple-mentation. In this case, the cost of the system and the cost of oper-ating it are relatively low. On the other hand, the firm misses out on business opportunities because of lack of capacity and allows competitors to enter the market. A situation of choosing a resource constraint is appropriate for firms that have a critical and expensive resource whose capacity is difficult to increase, that presents a strate-gic advantage to the organization, and is one of its core competen-cies. If, indeed, the decision is to have the constraint a resource constraint, the constraint should be in the most critical or most expensive resource in the system.

The question of where the constraint should be leads to an equally important question: Where should the constraint not be? In today's competitive market, in most cases, the constraint should not be in operations. We should not reach the point where operations are the system constraint. Operations are a function that can usually be expanded or some of its tasks given to subcontractors. When production is a standard process, operations should not be a system constraint. The role of the head of operations in a business firm is to make operations transparent to decision makers—that is, operations will see to it that the needed quantities will be produced at the predetermined timetables and at the required quality. Operations will thus contribute their share to strategy and the business success of the firm. Good and effective operations are a complex and complicated issue, and "transparency" for decision makers is difficult. To achieve this, operations should have protective capacity and may occasionally be at excess capacity. Production plants in Japan realized this from accumulated experience, and they are designing their production lines with an excess capacity of about 30 percent. It is clear that protective capacity is just one way to create transparent operations. The appropriate use of the managerial approaches described in earlier chapters is a necessary condition for achieving a situation where operations are not a system constraint.

The advantages of a market constraint (excess capacity) are the disadvantage of being in a state of resource constraints: an organization with excess capacity does not give up on orders and on possibilities for increasing output. This has strategic importance: giving up market share because of a resource constraint allows competitors to enter the market, which poses a threat to the organization in the long run. Excess capacity can also help the firm deal with occasional demands, large contracts, and emerging market opportunities.

Having a market constraint carries a higher price tag because the investment in resources costs more. Being a market constraint is more appropriate for organizations where resource costs are not large.

An organization must also examine whether research and development and marketing and sales are indeed permanent bottlenecks. In situations where these departments are not bottlenecks, the causes should be examined at the strategic and tactical levels.

Chapter Summary

Sales and marketing personnel are a permanent bottleneck in an organization. To increase their output, we must deal with their efficiency and effectiveness. The sales force can be made more efficient by reducing their noneffective time. Effectiveness is increased by focusing on high-potential customers through strategic gating. The seven steps of management by constraints, in addition to product differentiation and market segmentation, can increase the contribution of sales and enhance the value of an organization.

7

Focused Current Reality Tree

- Appreciate how many undesirable effects are caused by a few core problems.

A current reality tree (CRT) is a novel focusing tool based on logical thinking (Goldratt, 1994; Dettmer, 1998). The tool is used to identify the core problems in the organization. The underlying assumption is that the organization has a few core problems, and most of the other problems are symptoms of the core problems. If we solve the core problems, then many of the other problems will be solved as well. The objectives of the tool are as follows:

- To identify the core problems of the organization, the system, or subsystem

- To deepen the understanding that every system has a *small* number of core problems and that they are the cause of *most* problems

- To establish communication channels among managers in the organization

When a patient goes to his or her physician for a checkup and complains about various symptoms (headaches, perspiration, high fever), a good physician will try to find the "core problems" of the patient and to treat them.

Focused current reality tree (fCRT): A graphic managerial tool for helping identify the core problems of the system or organization.

A graph of a focused current reality tree is depicted as a logical tree describing cause-effect relations among the problems of the organization. A template for a fCRT is given in Figure 7.1.

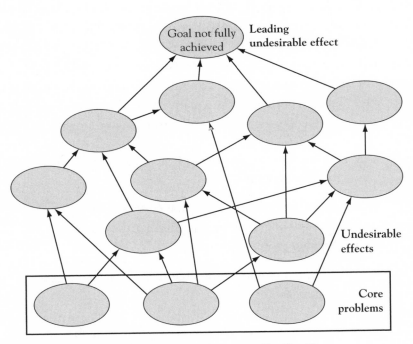

Figure 7.1. Template for a Focused Current Reality Tree.

Using an fCRT

An fCRT is a powerful tool that identifies the organization's core problems. Constructing an fCRT requires attention to several specific matters.

Principles of Constructing an fCRT

An fCRT can be constructed by a single manager or by a team. Because the tool is a subjective one and an organization's problems look different from different perspectives, it is better to have a team of managers and workers construct the fCRT. Occasionally an outside consulting group called in to diagnose the organization's problems constructs the fCRT.

Information Sources

The following are information sources for constructing an fCRT:

- Personal knowledge of managers and workers

- Interviews with managers and workers

- Review of the firm's or organization's sites

- Balance sheets, marketing reports, operations reports, and other reports in the organization

- Customers and suppliers

List of Undesirable Effects

For a phenomenon to be considered an *undesirable effect* (UDE) and to be included in the fCRT, three conditions must be satisfied:

1. The phenomenon must exist.

2. The phenomenon must be undesirable.

3. The phenomenon must be under our control or influence.

The third condition is especially important. A statement like "the weather is too cold" (and therefore more patients are expected in the emergency department) will not enter the analysis as a UDE because we have no control over the weather and cannot influence it.

On the other hand, there are phenomena beyond our control, but we do influence them. For example, "many customers leave the HMO" is a legitimate UDE. Competition is a predominant factor affecting abandonment, but we also have a strong influence on customer abandonment. UDEs will always be written as *negative* statements.

The "Leading Undesirable Effect"

The list of UDEs will always include the leading one, which is that we are not achieving the goal. In business organizations, the leading undesirable effect will be expressed as "the value of the firm is not sufficiently enhanced." In other organizations, the leading UDE could simply be "goal not fully achieved." For example, the chief medical director of a hospital can list the leading UDE as "the number of hospital deaths is too high."

All UDEs in an fCRT will relate, directly or indirectly, to the leading undesirable effect. Such an effect means that it contributes to the leading UDE of not achieving the goal.

Focusing on the Important Undesirable Effects

For the analysis using the fCRT to be simple and fast, we should limit our focus to eight to fourteen UDEs. After brainstorming, interviews, and examination of documents and reports, many more UDEs are suggested. The number of UDEs can be reduced in one of two ways: combining similar UDEs under one UDE or deleting UDEs that are less important relative to others on the list.

Finding Logical Relations Among Undesirable Effects

One type of logical relation among undesirable effects is a *cause-effect relation*. This will be depicted as an arrow leading from one UDE that is the cause to another that is the effect. Figure 7.2

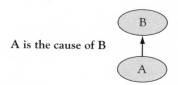

A is the cause of B

Figure 7.2. Cause-Effect Relation Between Undesirable Effects.

describes graphically a causal relation between two UDEs. An example of a cause-effect relation is shown in Figure 7.3.

An "extensive *or*" relation is presented in Figure 7.4. When an "extensive *or*" relationship exists and when both undesirable effects A and B exist, a third resulting undesirable effect is much more severe. An example is presented in Figure 7.5.

When the price is higher than competitors' prices, customers abandon. When the performance of the product is inferior, customers

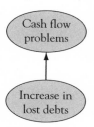

Figure 7.3. Example of a Cause-Effect Relation Between Undesirable Effects.

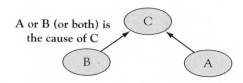

A or B (or both) is the cause of C

Figure 7.4. An "Extensive *Or*" Logical Relation.

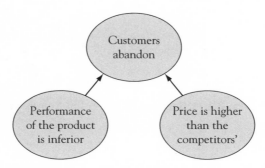

Figure 7.5. Example of an "Extensive *Or*" Logical Relation of Undesirable Effects.

abandon. If both UDEs happen (high price and poor performance), more customers abandon the system (see Figure 7.6).

The advantage of identifying such a "logical *and*" relation is that it is enough to solve either problem A or problem B to avoid problem C. There is no need to deal with both A and B. As shown in Figure 7.7, the contribution volume dropped as a result of combining two UDEs simultaneously. It is enough to deal with one of these UDEs to solve the problem of decreasing contribution volume.

In a "loop relation" (see Figure 7.8), A is the cause of B, B is the cause of C, and C is the cause of A. An example of such a relation is presented in Figure 7.9.

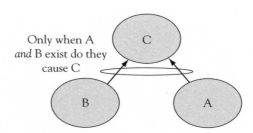

Figure 7.6. A "Logical *And*" Relation of Undesirable Effects.

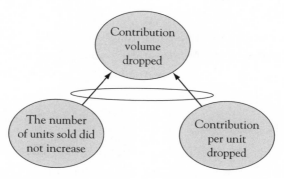

Figure 7.7. Example of a "Logical *And*" Relation.

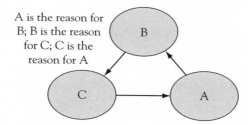

Figure 7.8. A Logical Loop Relation.

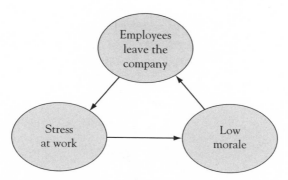

Figure 7.9. Example of a Loop Relation Between Undesirable Effects.

Inferences

Inferences are explanations or conclusions and insights that were not included in the list of undesirable effects. These are usually logical relations that explain nontrivial relations among problems. In Figure 7.10, the relation is drawn as a rectangle.

Constructing an fCRT

Construction of the fCRT begins with the leading undesirable effect. Under this effect, we will position all the problems that were identified as causes linked directly to the leading undesirable effect, and they are linked with cause-effect arrows. We add, layer by layer, the UDEs that are causes for the previously included UDEs. As needed, we add inferences that explain nontrivial relations among UDEs and insights learned during the tree construction. At the end of the process, we have at the bottom of the tree a small number of problems that have no other UDEs that explain them. These are the core problems.

Identifying Core Problems

The small number of core problems left at the end of constructing the fCRT could be UDEs or effects that we infer to be core problems. Usually there are only three or fewer. If we end up with a large

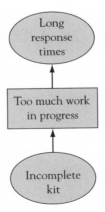

Figure 7.10. Example of Inference.

number of UDEs at the bottom of the tree, we try to think of a factor or issue that could be the cause of many of the problems or possibly one of the core problems. This inferred UDE is listed under the previous problems, linked to them by causal links, and it will be the real core problem. Core problems can therefore be UDEs or inferences (conclusions of the team constructing the fCRT). The following are examples of core problems in organizations:

- A manager or management that is too centralized

- Lack of a clear strategy

- Unstructured processes

- Inappropriate performance measures

- Lack of focus

- A company driven by technological thinking rather than business thinking

- Gap between professional and managerial abilities

Exercising Orthogonal Control

Orthogonal control is an independent identification of core problems. After the core problems have been identified, we must ask the question, If we solve the core problems, will the leading undesirable effect significantly change? For example, a core problem in an fCRT was identified as "lack of focus." Will solving this problem significantly enhance the value of the firm? If the answer is yes, this is indeed a core problem, and it must be dealt with. If not, the tree should be reexamined. Figure 7.11 shows a typical fCRT.

Advantages and disadvantages of using an fCRT

The advantages of using an fCRT are the simplicity of the tool and the focusing directed at core problems. The tool enables better communication within the organization and differentiating between a symptom (undesirable effect) and a core problem.

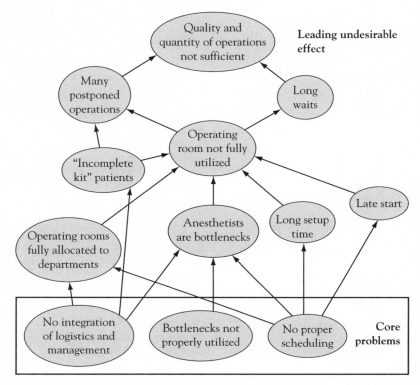

Figure 7.11. Example of an fCRT.

A disadvantage of an fCRT is its being a subjective tool. This disadvantage can be reduced by having a team construct it, especially if the team is interdisciplinary. Orthogonal control also helps diminish this disadvantage.

Routine Use of an fCRT

1. Collect information about the problems in the organization (personal knowledge of managers, interviews with managers and workers, site visits, reports and documents, interviews with customers and suppliers).

2. Articulate the leading UDE of the organization. In a business organization, this is "value enhancement of the organization is insufficient." In other organizations, one must determine the organizational goal and accordingly the leading UDE.

3. List the main UDEs (eight to fourteen problems).

4. Arrange the UDEs in cause-effect relations where the leading UDE is at the top.

5. Identify the core problems of the organization or unit (not more than three).

6. Apply orthogonal control. Ask yourself, "Will solving each of the identified core problems significantly improve the leading undesirable effect?"

7. Make a list of action items that will deal with the core problems. Use a focusing table and a focusing matrix.

Chapter Summary

An fCRT is a simple tool for detecting the core problems of an organization. This tool provides the insight that the organization has only a small number of core problems, and solving them will enhance the value of the organization. The fCRT also serves as a communication tool within the organization. Because this is a subjective tool, it is recommended that it be constructed by an interdisciplinary team.

8

Resolving Managerial Conflicts

Objective

- Understand the nature of managerial conflicts and how to resolve them in mutually beneficial ways

Dictionaries define conflict as "a prolonged struggle," "a trial of strength," or "strong disagreement." We focus on those managerial conflicts where the opposing alternatives have a common goal. The following are some examples:

- *Decentralization versus centralization*—for example, centralization of management within a health maintenance organization (HMO) versus decentralization of management to individual clinics
- *A large variety of services or products versus a limited number*—for example, a center for women's health may offer comprehensive health care services versus only gynecological ones
- *Keeping large versus small inventories*
- *Developing a generic future product versus developing a specific product requested by a customer*
- *Opposing policies*—for example, in the emergency department of a hospital, a policy of comprehensive medical testing versus a policy of quick decisions on admission or discharge

---

Conflict: a clash between two alternative actions that
have a common goal

We use the following three-step method to deal with managerial conflicts:

1. Describe the conflict with a conflict resolution diagram
   (CRD) (Goldratt, 1994).
2. Solve the conflict by challenging the assumptions on the
   CRD with the following approaches:
   - Differentiation
   - Globalization
   - Breaking assumptions
3. Create actions for implementation based on the challenged
   assumptions.

Let us consider, for example, a situation involving a basket of
services. An HMO is considering offering a large basket of services,
procedures, and medications versus offering a limited variety. Each
alternative has its own advantages. Offering a large variety can
improve contribution and enhance the value of the HMO. Offering only a limited variety allows for focusing, specialization, and cost
reduction. Both alternative actions create value for the HMO. The
common goal, of course, is value enhancement.

A conflict is sometimes dealt with erroneously by searching for a
compromise using various optimization techniques. In the above
example, an optimization tool may suggest an "exact" optimal solution of offering seventeen specified services and procedures. Using
such a solution will cause the loss of the advantage of diversification with a large variety and the advantages of focusing and quality achieved with a small variety. The suggested method solves
conflicts in one of two ways (see Figure 8.1):

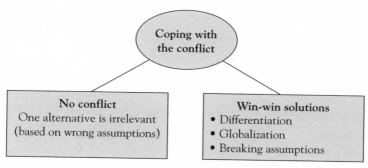

Figure 8.1. Dealing with Conflicts.

1. Generate a solution that will preserve most of the advantages of each alternative and will reduce the disadvantages of each. This is a "win-win" approach. It can be achieved through differentiation, globalization, and breaking of assumptions. Identifying such situations is not assured, but experience shows that it is frequently possible.

2. Present one alternative as irrelevant because it is based on wrong assumptions. Hence, there is no real conflict.

Steps in Dealing with Managerial Conflicts

The graphic representation of a CRD is the first and most important step of conflict resolution, as it crystallizes the elements of the conflict. The second step is methodically to resolve the conflict.

Drawing a CRD

The CRD is an important communication tool to present conflicts and try to solve them. The following elements appear in a CRD:

- The goal of the system or subsystem

- The two alternatives that create the conflict

- The advantages of each alternative or the need for each, based on the system's goal

The various elements shown in Figure 8.2 are logically linked: arrows 1, 2, 3, and 4 represent conditional relations, and arrow 5 depicts the alleged impossibility of simultaneously satisfying both alternatives.

The assumptions in the CRD are as follows:

1. The advantages of alternative A contribute to achieving the goal.

2. The advantages of alternative B contribute to achieving the goal.

3. Action based on alternative A brings the advantages for achieving the goal.

4. Action based on alternative B brings the advantages for achieving the goal.

5. Alternatives A and B cannot be acted on simultaneously.

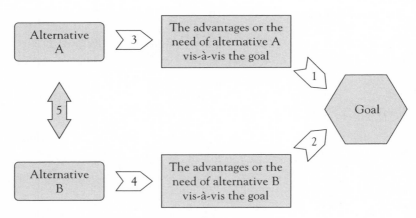

Figure 8.2. A Conflict Resolution Diagram.

The CRD of the HMO variety of service example is presented in Figure 8.3.

Conflict Resolution

We now demonstrate conflict resolution using differentiation, globalization, and breaking of assumptions.

Differentiation

Using the differentiation mechanism, a Pareto analysis of the various services shows that 20 percent of services accounts for 80 percent of the HMO's profits. The inclination is to offer the HMO members the entire variety of services. However, the services of group A in the Pareto analysis will be provided by the HMO itself whereas group B and C services will be provided through a subcontractor.

Globalization

Globalization is demonstrated by the following example. A large public organization has to renew its fleet of cars. The conflict is whether to buy cheaper cars or more expensive and reliable ones (see Figure 8.4). When we look at the car purchases from a global

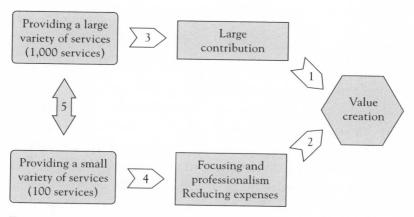

Figure 8.3. A CRD for Service Variety.

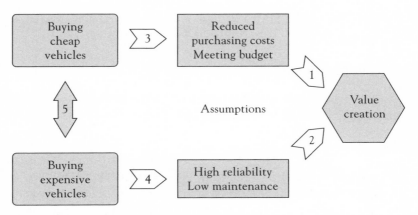

Figure 8.4. A CRD for the Car Fleet Example.

perspective, we should assess the life-cycle cost (LCC) of the fleet. This is an expansion of globalization over time. Analysis shows that from the LCC perspective, buying the expensive cars is actually cheaper. The maintenance and fuel costs, given the high mileage these cars are expected to drive, make the purchase price only a small part of the LCC. The budget-constraint problem was also resolved by agreeing to spread the purchase price over a period of several years. In this example, the alternative of buying the cheap cars is actually irrelevant, and thus there is no conflict.

Breaking Assumptions

The mechanism for breaking assumptions checks the assumptions that exist in every CRD. We demonstrate this mechanism using the following example. The development department of a medical software firm is developing a special version of a computerized patient record for a specific HMO. The conflict that brought about a heated discussion in the weekly management meeting was, "Should we start development immediately, or should we first spend time to define the project in an orderly and structured manner?" (see Figure 8.5). The assumptions at the basis of this conflict are as follows:

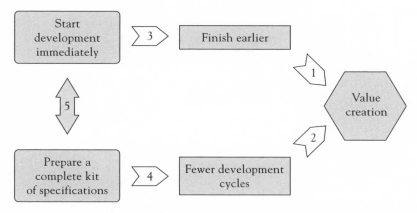

Figure 8.5. A CRD for the Software Development Example.

1. An early completion of the project enhances the value of the firm.

2. Development in fewer cycles enhances the value of the firm.

3. If we start the project earlier, we will finish it earlier.

4. If we provide orderly definitions for requested changes and the different requirements of the customer, development can be done in fewer development cycles.

5. It is not possible to start immediate development simultaneously with providing complete definitions in a structured manner.

To demonstrate that one of the alternatives is not relevant, we will try to break the weakest assumption, which is assumption 3. It is clear that an earlier start of the project does not necessarily translate to an earlier completion. If this is the case, the top alternative ("start immediately") is actually irrelevant, and the bottom one should be chosen.

Resolving a conflict by breaking an assumption is called *injection*. The injection is added to the CRD, as shown in Figure 8.6. Figures 8.7 through 8.14 present some common conflicts in health care organizations.

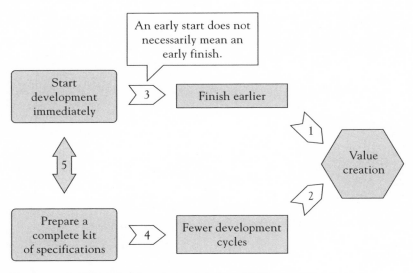

Figure 8.6. Example of an Injection in a CRD.

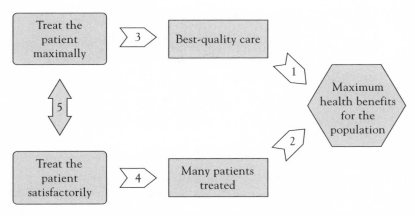

Figure 8.7. A Public Hospital Outpatient Clinic with the Conflict of Treating Maximally Versus Treating Satisfactorily.

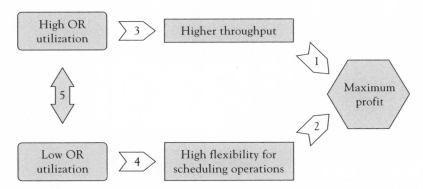

Figure 8.8. A Private Hospital Operating Room (OR) Scheduling Conflict of Volume Versus Flexibility.

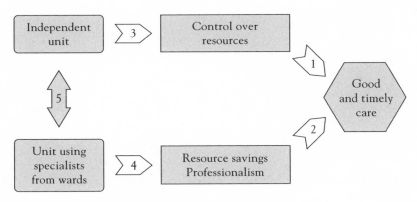

Figure 8.9. Conflict in an Emergency Department (1).

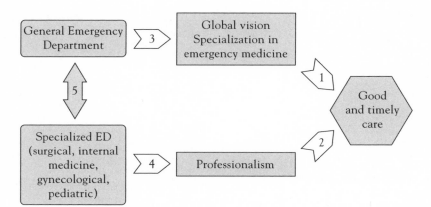

Figure 8.10. Conflict in an Emergency Department (2).

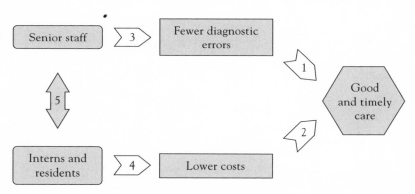

Figure 8.11. Conflict of Errors Versus Cost in an Emergency Department.

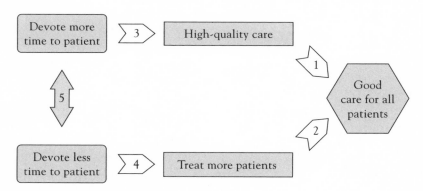

Figure 8.12. Clinical Conflict in Diagnosis.

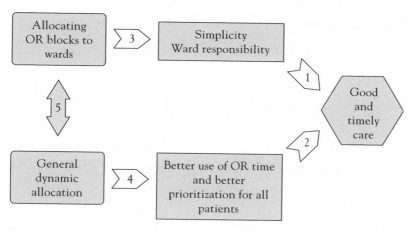

Figure 8.13. Conflict in an OR: What to Do with Patients.

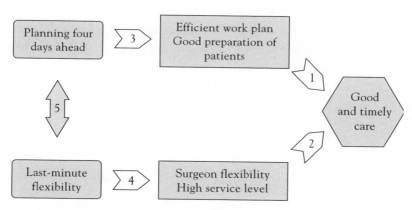

Figure 8.14. Flexibility Conflict in OR Scheduling.

Routine Use of the Conflict Resolution Approach

1. Define the goal of the system or subsystem.
2. Display the conflict in a CRD.
3. Try to resolve the conflict by differentiation, globalization, or breaking of assumptions.
4. When breaking assumptions, add the injections to the CRD.
5. Make a list of action items that will resolve the conflict. Use a focusing table and focusing matrix.

Chapter Summary

Managerial conflicts are seemingly contradictory alternatives with a common objective function. Many conflicts can be resolved either through win-win solutions or by concluding that one alternative is irrelevant. Conflicts are resolved through displaying the conflict on a CRD and analyzing the CRD using differentiation, globalization, and breaking of assumptions.

9

The Efficiencies Syndrome

Objective

- Learn what the human aspects of the "efficiencies syndrome" are, its negative effects, and how to avoid it

In previous chapters, we have seen that the bottlenecks, the critical resources of an organization, must be exploited. The other resources must be subordinated to the constraint. Experience has shown that the management of noncritical resources of an organization is usually associated with a painful policy failure (policy constraint) known as the *efficiencies syndrome* (Goldratt and Cox, 1992). This situation is common among managers and workers of all types of organizations (service, industry, health, development, and not-for-profit).

The Efficiencies Syndrome

The efficiencies syndrome is illustrated by the 1-2-3 process in Figure 9.1. It is clear that under current conditions, the output of this process is fifty units per day, and the (capacity) utilization of the resources of the three departments in the figure is 50 percent, 100 percent, and 67 percent, respectively.

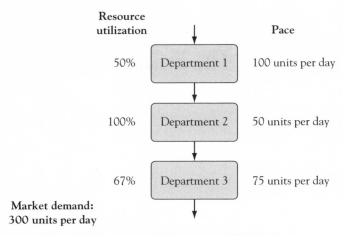

Figure 9.1. A 1-2-3 Process and Department Utilization.

Efficiencies syndrome: A situation where there is a desire to operate the noncritical resources more than is needed or emphasizing utilization of inputs rather than focusing on outputs.

What will happen if the system is measured by the "average resource utilization," which is 72 percent? To increase the average utilization, workers in department 1 will try to achieve a maximal resource use of 100 percent. As a result, the average utilization will increase to 90 percent. In department 3, they will also try to increase use to 100 percent, but they are limited by what department 2 (the bottleneck) supplies them.

Even though the measure of average resource utilization has increased, the system output has not. On the other hand, exploiting the other resources may result in the following undesirable effects on the system:

- People working harder without increasing effective output

- Deterioration of control of what is important

- Decrease in the quality of decisions

- Increase in the amount of work in process

- Wasting of resources (personnel and equipment)

- Increase in expenditures

- Decrease in output

- A feeling of working harder with declining output, leading to loss of confidence in management

The efficiencies syndrome results from behavior of managers and workers, such as the following:

- Western cultural views of idle persons as being lazy, meaning one must work or at least appear to be working

- Fear of being transferred or laid off

- Lack of a global vision and a belief that fully utilizing resources contributes to achieving the goal

- Lack of distinction between critical resources (bottle-necks) and noncritical resources (with excess capacity)

- Feeling that purchasing equipment or hiring personnel must be justified

- Measuring systems by inputs (as reflected in local incentives and bonuses)

- Measuring systems by "resource utilization"

- Desire to look important and busy

In the customer service department of a hospital, there was a need for another computer for a newly hired data entry operator. Management declined the request on the grounds that the utilization of the other computers is low and that several operators can share a computer. The result was that one of the operators spent time writing an application that duplicates files, just to increase the capacity utilization of the computers in the hope of justifying the need for another one.

A worker in a firm told the following story: "In the morning, we throw the garbage from the garbage cans onto the floor and start sweeping the floor. When the boss arrives, he sees that we are busy."

A large organization experienced the "fluorescent lights effect." All the workers were eager to show that they work late. The office lights were on until the late hours of the evening, even when the workers were not there. The hours of lighted offices were a measure of workers' diligence and their importance to the system. In this organization, it was known that some of the managers would call their subordinates' offices at very late hours, without any necessity, just so they would know that the boss might be looking for them late.

In a not-for-profit organization, all meetings begin at 10:00 P.M. because before that everybody is "busy."

In a high-tech organization, management decided to evaluate the capacity utilization of newly purchased equipment. They generated comparative data on utilization on similar machines in various departments. As a result, workers kept the engines of the machines running even during calibration, resulting in eventual serious damage to some machines.

In a newly created start-up firm, everybody works from early morning to late night because this is the customary culture in similar companies.

The efficiencies syndrome is responsible for stretching time and the "drawer effect" where workers make sure they have some work to do at times of trouble (when they have to justify their existence).

In the repair shop of instruments in a hospital, technicians always leave aside a few defective instruments before trying to diagnose their problems. They use this ploy for keeping busy on days when they do not have other repairs.

Dealing with the Efficiencies Syndrome

The failure of the efficiencies syndrome is clear and is an example of system chaos. This phenomenon does not exist with individuals outside of their work environment; nobody judges their car by its utilization but rather by its effectiveness. People do not expect their computers to work all the time.

We must shift our orientation to measuring throughput and learn to live with the fact that noncritical resources may be idle some of the time, especially if they want to be able to achieve fast response times.

The following are some things workers could do during idle times:

- Flexible training and self-learning

- Activities for process improvement and quality management

- Help at bottlenecks

- Shift work from the bottleneck departments to less busy departments

- Preventive maintenance

From a global perspective, a product or service line does not have to be balanced in its capacity. The line contains different resources, some cheap, some expensive. It is not expected that the capacity utilization of the clerical or cleaning staff in a clinic will be the same as the capacity utilization of expensive resources like physicians and nurses. It is inconceivable that an inexpensive worker will be a bottleneck and will bring the whole system to a halt. Hence, line balancing does not stand the test of reality. Because of fluctuations, there is an extra motivation to create some excess capacity in some resources, as is discussed further in Chapter 14.

However, the existence of excess capacity in the system, which is positive for the system and its throughput, could be a failure if the system people contract the efficiencies syndrome. This could lead to non-bottleneck resources becoming system constraints. A good manager should be able to deal with the efficiencies syndrome and find appropriate solutions. It is not easy to deal with this syndrome, and it requires a common language and a common managerial approach for managers and employees.

Chapter Summary

The efficiencies syndrome causes human resources and equipment to work more than necessary. This syndrome is fueled by managerial and cultural factors. The desire to show that one is busy, taking a local perspective and inappropriate measurement, all lead to enhancing this syndrome. Resolving the syndrome requires a change in organizational thinking, which is not easy to bring about.

10

The Evils of Long Response Times

Objective

- Understand the many negative effects of long response times and high levels of work in process

Long response times for service, production, and development processes are a major concern in today's management world. To find ways to shorten response times, we examine in this chapter the relation between response time and the amount of work in process (WIP).

Types of Inventories

The management of physical inventories (hardware, components, materials, documents, files, and the like) and nonphysical and human ones (development of software, business information in processing, patients hospitalized or waiting for tests, customers waiting in a bank, and so forth) plays an important role in business systems, operational systems, health care systems, and systems that are not for profit.

Three types of inventories are shown in Figure 10.1.

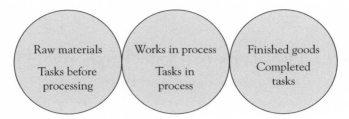

Figure 10.1. Types of Inventories.

Raw materials: Materials, components, information, tasks, and the like before they enter processing in the system; tasks that have not yet been handled.

Works in process: Intermediate products or tasks whose handling has been started but not yet completed; tasks in process.

The following are examples of WIP:

- Patients being treated in an emergency department (ED)

- Development of software and hardware that has not yet been completed

- Assemblies on an assembly line

- Purchase orders in the negotiating process or in the stage of approval

- Receipts handled in the accounting department

- Business information processing

- Equipment and instruments being repaired in the maintenance department

---

Finished goods: products, information, and tasks whose processing has been completed; completed missions.

Note that in this chapter, we focus only on WIP. Methods of managing WIP are different from those for managing raw materials or finished goods. Applying the tools for WIP management to other inventory types can harm the organization.

The Evils of WIP

Figure 10.2 presents two imaging and testing centers of two competing health maintenance organizations (HMOs). The clinics are similar and perform identical functions. This example can be relevant for many types of organizations. Both testing centers operate in the same market and have similar resources and capabilities. Both the arrival and the departure rates in each center are twenty patients per hour. The difference between the two centers is the

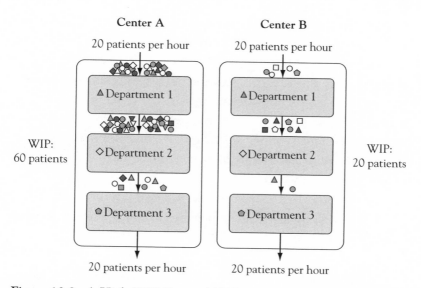

Figure 10.2. A High-WIP Center (A) Versus a Low-WIP Center (B).

amount of WIP: center A has sixty patients in the system, and center B has twenty patients. These numbers include patients being seen or treated in each department and patients waiting before each department. Let us ignore for the moment the reasons causing the difference in the amount of WIP between the two centers and focus on the question of whether the higher level of WIP in center A improves or harms this center's performance.

Relation Between Response Time and Level of WIP

High levels of WIP lead to long response times, and the average response time of the system is proportional to the WIP level. The average time spent by a patient in center A of Figure 10.2 is three hours compared with one hour in center B. The number of patients waiting in center A is sixty compared with twenty in center B. On the average, the throughput time (time from entry until departure) of a patient arriving in center A will be three hours ($60 \div 20 = 3$), whereas it will be only one hour in center B ($20 \div 20 = 1$).

The average response time of the process equals the WIP divided by the system throughput rate. This is one of the Little formulas of queuing theory. It can be shown that this is true for any queue discipline (first in, first out; last in, first out; and so forth) (see Hillier and Lieberman, 2002).

Let us now examine the gross and net response times of the system. In the majority of situations, most of the response time will be caused by the waiting times at the various workstations. Treatment or processing time is rather short. Several studies on response times in various service and industry organizations show that the net processing time is only 5 to 10 percent of the total response time. Our experience shows that in many cases, *work time is no more than 1 percent of total response time*. The following examples demonstrate this surprising ratio:

- The average gross time for a patient in a hospital ED is about four hours. The total net treatment time is only a few minutes.

- A purchase request for an item from the request initiation until the order is sent to the supplier takes several days (gross time). The actual time spent by the purchasing people on the request at the various workstations barely exceeds one hour.
- The process of approving a loan or a mortgage takes several days whereas the actual net time spent on the forms is no longer than two hours.
- The response time of a subcontractor for fixing a medical instrument is up to two weeks. The net time spent fixing the instrument is in the magnitude of two hours or less.

The *gross response time (throughput time)* of the process equals the sum of *processing times (net times)* of the individual unit (patient) in the various stations plus the sum of the *waiting times* of the unit (patient) before the various stations.

The *response time of a process* is proportional to the *amount of WIP*. If the amount of WIP is reduced, the response time will be reduced.

Evils of excessive WIP: The damage to the performance of the organization caused by high levels of WIP. These are the undesirable consequences of high levels of WIP.

Undesirable consequences of a long response time: The damage to the performance of the organization caused by its long response time.

Because response time is proportional to the amount of WIP, the undesirable consequences of a long response time are identical to those of WIP. These are listed below.

Reduction in Throughput

Windows of opportunity for new services or products open for only short periods. An organization with fast response times (for submitting proposals, development, production, arranging business plans, and the like) can take advantage of these opportunities. Furthermore, the faster an organization comes out with new services or products and the shorter the response times for committing these to customers, the higher the prices they can charge. Innovative products that reach the market fast and ahead of competitors can occasionally attract the best customers in the market. There are also situations where being first to market enables an organization to capture a significant market share, making it difficult for competitors to penetrate the market.

High Operating Expenses

Accumulation of WIP and long response times lead to high operating expenses (inventory carrying costs, maintenance and control) and additional financial consequences.

Diminished Quality

The longer the response time and the longer work is in process, the more the damage to quality. Two reasons account for this:

1. Materials that had been delayed in the process are left unprotected and vulnerable to environmental, physical, mechanical, and other damages. In service units or with information technology, the quality of decisions and of treatment diminish because of the long time that has passed from the beginning of processing until the end. This is especially true if several employees take part in the process.

2. The longer the response time, feedback on earlier mistakes arrives later to the station responsible for the mistake. The lack of immediate feedback creates more errors.

The longer a patient spends in the hospital or in a clinic, the more the patient is exposed to contracting infections.

A claims case receives inferior treatment the longer it stays as WIP. This is due to piling up of nonrelevant papers, distraction by other files, and the changing of treating hands.

The quality of an insurance claim decision or a court decision diminishes when the claim is handled by many people or many judges.

Diminished Control

The piling up of WIP allows workers degrees of freedom in selecting preferred tasks to work on. As a result, the control that managers have diminishes as well as their ability to dictate priorities. Reducing the amount of WIP allows better and more effective control.

Diminished Flexibility to Market and Technological Changes

Long response times and accumulating WIP make it difficult to introduce changes in services or products. Such changes are needed if market preferences change or there is a need for an engineering change. Occasionally there is a need to trash the entire WIP, especially if there is pressure for immediate introduction of a new product into the market. In other situations where costs accumulated due to high levels of WIP, there is a temptation to wait with the needed changes until some inventory is consumed. This may lead to missed windows of opportunity.

Diminished Cash Flow

A company needs return capital to finance the WIP. Companies with slow response times and large inventories may face a crisis caused by unfavorable cash flow. They are usually required to pay for raw materials within a short time, whereas payment will be received later because of the long response time.

Diminished Motivation of Managers and Workers

Managers and workers operating in a high WIP environment with long response times experience frustration resulting from work pressure and frequent shifting from task to task. Facing a continuous situation of not being able to achieve the desired throughput and the temporary frustration from not meeting timetables diminishes the motivation of workers and management.

Missed Deadlines

The accumulation of WIP and long response times diminish an organization's ability to meet deadlines and adhere to timetables.

Lack of Customer Satisfaction

The service, treatment, or products that are delivered late or with inferior quality create customer dissatisfaction. This can lead to a loss of customers.

Diminished Forecasting Capability

Forecasting is important to organizations for planning the human resources, raw materials inventory, developing marketing and sales channels, and cash flow. Forecasting ability is a function of the forecasting horizon. The relation between the quality of forecasts and the forecasting horizon is presented in Figure 10.3 (Goldratt and Fox, 1986).

Improving forecasting ability through the use of analytical and marketing tools can help the organization to some extent. However, reducing system response times will significantly improve forecasting ability. If the system response time is t_2 (days or weeks), then one must forecast the market demand at that time. If the response time is reduced to t_1, the quality of forecasting market demand will improve dramatically. Reduced response time, among other benefits, will be achieved by reducing WIP.

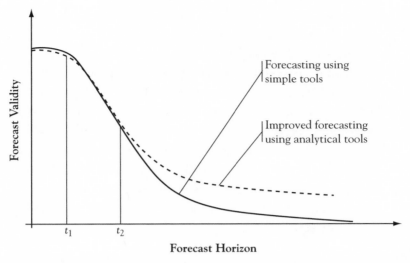

Figure 10.3. Effect of the Forecasting Horizon on Forecasting Quality.

Diminished Throughput

High levels of WIP cause system inefficiency, which diminishes throughput. Work that comes in and out of a bottleneck can make the bottleneck ineffective. Jobs that enter the bottleneck at inappropriate times because of lack of control also diminish system throughput.

Acquired Infections

In hospitals, clinics, and nursing homes, long response times result in high WIP. The longer patients stay in a medical environment and the more patients who are there at any given time increase dramatically the chance of acquiring a host of infections, leading to additional morbidity, costs, and mortality, along with diminished quality of life.

A firm specializing in advanced medical testing equipment won an international contract worth millions of dollars. The performance of the firm was characterized by delays in delivering orders, high production costs, many rejections in quality control and by customers, and problems with management and control. They tried to remedy the situation by introducing technological changes, but to no avail. They also considered introducing a sophisticated information system. A careful analysis of the situation revealed a large amount of WIP, resulting in long response times. Some components in the WIP inventory when exposed too long to oxygen resulted in excessive oxygenation that in turn caused component and equipment failure. Once the WIP inventory and response times were reduced, the firm proceeded to produce at high throughput and with near zero failures, to the full satisfaction of customers.

An insurance company offered supplementary health insurance to members of HMOs. The response time for generating policies was about six weeks from the date the customer signed the request form until the policy went into effect. During this long time period, many potential customers cancelled their request. In addition, many files piled up in the office, causing pressure on employees, which resulted in mistakes in writing up and approving policies. Some of these mistakes were a result of the file being handled by several different people over the course of several weeks. The reduction of WIP and the resulting reduction in response time yielded higher quality, and the number of cancelled requests dropped dramatically. This enabled management to focus on the more important issues in the firm, those relating to marketing (see Eden and Ronen, 1993).

In a medical staffing firm, the process of assigning workers to hospitals was long. As a result, many potential workers simply disappeared from the scene as they managed to find assignments on their own or through other agencies. This situation is sometimes referred to as *evaporating inventory*. Shortening the processing response time greatly improved the situation.

A community hospital reported a high rate of cross-infections in patients hospitalized in the internal medicine wards. A careful comparative analysis with other local hospitals revealed that this hospital had an average length of stay that was two days longer than others. Some of the causes for the excessive stay were administrative. The discharge policy required too many signatures, and the processing of information was also slow. Administrative policies were changed, resulting in an immediate reduction of 1.2 days in the length of stay. The number of cross-infections also dropped.

Causes of Excess WIP

Several policy constraints are responsible for the accumulation of WIP above what is required for efficient operation of the system. These are described below.

Efficiencies Syndrome

As a result of the efficiencies syndrome, which causes additional (unnecessary) work for noncritical resources, there is an excessive buildup of WIP inventory.

Viewing Inventory as Assets

Looking at an organization from the narrow perspective of financial accounting can wrongly encourage management to increase inventory to show larger assets on the balance sheet (Geri and Ronen, 2005). The adverse effects for the organization resulting from excessive WIP are greater than the seemingly negative effect of showing smaller inventories.

Ignorance

A knowledge gap in understanding the importance of WIP and not using methods to reduce WIP results in excessive WIP.

Chapter Summary

The undesirable consequences of long response times, which are those of WIP, are responsible for diminished work quality and customer satisfaction. There is also a diminishment of throughput, control, and cash flow and the added expenses resulting from excessive inventories and excessive response times.

Shortening response time and reducing the level of WIP serve as a leverage for significant improvements in organizational performance and enhancing its value (see Figure 10.4). The methods for reducing the volume of WIP and shortening response time are detailed in Chapter 11.

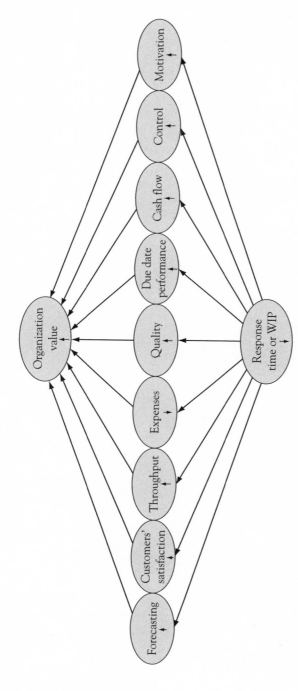

Figure 10.4. Effect of Reducing WIP on Organization Function and Value.

11

Reducing Response Times

Objective

- Acquire practical ways to substantially reduce
response times

Short response times have strategic and tactical importance.
They serve as a strategic value driver for an organization. At the
strategic level, short response times allow an organization flexibility
in moving from one product to another, from one service to another,
and from one product or service line to another to better respond to
market changes. In a changing market, with its inherent uncertainty,
a flexible organization can adapt itself quickly to changes in the environment and increase its chances of survival and success.

At the tactical level, fast response times enable an organization,
as we have seen in the previous chapter, to work with low levels of
work in process (WIP), reduce costs, and increase throughput.

Methods for Reducing WIP and Response Time

Both response times and the amount of WIP can be reduced by various methods. We will first list them and then expand and demonstrate them.

- Strategic gating (discussed in Chapter 5)

- Tactical gating (discussed in Chapter 5)

- Working with a complete kit

- Managing the bottlenecks (discussed in Chapter 5)

- Working by just-in-time (JIT) rule I

- Working by JIT rule II

    Working with small and appropriate work batches
    and work packages

    Working with small transfer batches

- Working by JIT rule III

- Measurement and control

- Implementing the drum-buffer-rope (DBR) mechanism (discussed in Chapter 5)

- Quality improvement and reduction of the "garbage plant" in the process

- Avoiding bad multitasking

- Implementing group technology

- Working in parallel rather than serially

Strategic Gating

Strategic gating, as discussed in Chapter 5, is a managerial tool that screens out tasks that should not reach the system and thus not consume the scarce time of the bottleneck. Organizations that routinely apply strategic gating, especially in areas of development (for example, pharmaceutical companies), marketing, and sales, reduce the workloads by up to 25 percent, hence reducing the response time for the important tasks. The time to market is also reduced, which in turn contributes to competitiveness.

There are situations where strategic gating is not relevant. For example, emergency departments (EDs) do not decide that some patients will not be admitted. Hospitals, especially private ones, do exercise strategic gating. A hospital may decide that certain types of surgery will not be performed. Many surgical centers are shying away from gynecological surgery because of frequent malpractice suits. Some hospitals specialize in specific procedures, thus screening out others. This is strategic gating.

Tactical Gating

Tactical gating, discussed in Chapter 5, is the controlled release of tasks into the system and is appropriate for all organizations. The tasks that pass the strategic-gating screening must go through tactical gating (Pass and Ronen, 2003). The roles of tactical gating are as follows:

- Releasing only tasks with a complete kit

- Releasing tasks in small and appropriate batches

- Assuring that all tasks are released by one source (the gater) that is responsible for the tactical gating. The timing of task release will be determined by the bottleneck capacity while maintaining an appropriate buffer in front of the bottleneck (for example, the DBR mechanism).

These roles are further detailed later in this chapter.

A good example of tactical gating is a triage nurse who sets priorities and channels patients to various destinations. EDs are divided into surgical emergencies, internal medicine, gynecology, and trauma.

Working with a Complete Kit

Working with a complete kit is one of the important principles in reducing response times. This principle, along with ways to implement it, is detailed in Chapter 12.

Managing Bottlenecks

The management-by-constraints approach for managing bottle-necks yields higher throughput on the one hand and reduced response time on the other. The contribution of the first two JIT rules to reducing response times is discussed below. Before we go into the details, we briefly present the JIT theory.

The JIT Method and Its Application in Health Care Systems

The JIT method is of utmost importance in reducing response times. It emerged from industrial plants in Japan and was also successfully used in service and health care organizations. About 70 percent of the success attributable to the JIT method is based on universal concepts and techniques that do not relate to the Japanese culture and have successfully been applied in Japan, the United States, and Europe. The remaining 30 percent contribution is culture-dependent and is not addressed in this book.

JIT is a method that stands on its own and can be applied as is. However, experience clearly demonstrates that the application outcomes are better when JIT is combined with other managerial approaches such as management by constraints, managing for quality, the complete kit concept, and others.

The JIT theory can be summarized by three basic and simple rules:

- Rule I: Work only as needed in terms of time, quantity, and specifications.

- Rule II: Work in small, appropriate, and smart batches.

- Rule III: Avoid waste and activities that do not add value to the organization.

JIT Rule I

This rule implies that a product or service should not be delivered earlier or later than the target time, one should not produce more than or less than the required quantity, and a product should be neither underdesigned nor overdesigned with regard to its specifications. This sounds so simple and obvious that one wonders what is new here.

JIT Rule I: Work only as needed in terms of time, quantity, and specifications.

We can identify two types of managerial deviations: shortage deviation and surplus deviation.

Shortage Deviation

Say demand is for ten units, and the actual supply is only eight. This is a serious deviation that interferes with supply to customers, interferes with cash flow, and damages reputation. However, such a deviation can be dealt with by routine control mechanisms of the organization and natural mechanisms that will usually close the gap, as follows:

- The worker, knowing that he or she will not meet demand, will meet the shortage within a short time.

- The worker's superior will monitor the demanded quantities and make sure the deviation is corrected.

- Sales and marketing managers will work to close the gap if others have not done so.

- The financial manager will point out situations with cash-flow gaps.

- The customer will approach management with a request to correct the deviation.

In other words, the organizational mechanism will work toward closing the gap.

Surplus Deviation

Say demand is for ten units, but twelve units have been provided. This deviation is usually not handled in the short term by the routine mechanisms of the organization and does not naturally generate feedback for workers and managers. Correction mechanisms are not triggered because of the following reasons:

- The worker feels that he or she is overachieving.

- Managers sometimes do not care about the surplus because they are busy handling crises elsewhere in the organization.

- Sales and marketing personnel have no knowledge about such a surplus.

- The financial manager will deal with this situation at the end of the year or, at best, at the end of a quarter. At that time, the accountants will become involved in how to write down the inventories.

- The customer may be totally unaware of surpluses.

Surplus deviations are not routinely dealt with even though they create much harm:

- If the resource is a bottleneck, then generating a surplus of two units (20 percent) translates into a 20 percent wastage of the resource. The entire system loses 20 percent of its throughput.

- Generating the surplus requires using materials and components beyond those planned for, thus inhibiting their use for other products.

- WIP is increased.

- It creates unneeded inventory.

In summary, being early may be as bad as being late. Similarly, overproducing may be as bad as underproducing. There is an effect of "double stealing" of bottleneck time and materials, causing bad planning and delays in supply. In addition, the increased WIP inventory brings about all the adverse consequences described in the previous chapter.

The bottom line of JIT rule I is that a surplus deviation is as bad as a shortage deviation.

Implementing JIT Rule I in Maintenance

The implementation of JIT rule I is useful and important for maintenance. The implications are that maintenance of equipment should not be done less than needed nor more than needed.

> In a large maintenance organization, one-third of labor hours was devoted to repairing equipment that was not in demand at the time of repair or that was not used at all (due to introduction of a new generation of equipment or having a surplus of a given equipment). As a result, the organization was late in many of the urgently needed repairs. Working in the spirit of JIT rule I resulted in a reduction in the number of early repairs and a total stoppage of unnecessary repairs. This reduced the backlog and improved meeting deadlines.

Implementing JIT Rule I in Scheduling of Tasks and Meetings

The following simple example demonstrates that JIT rule I with respect to timing is applicable to scheduling:

> A surgeon wants to start operating at 10:00 A.M. but tells the operating room (OR) staff that he wants everything ready at 9:30 A.M., the OR staff

requests that the patient be there at 9:00 A.M., and the nursing staff on the ward summons an orderly to transport the patient at 8:00 A.M.

Violating JIT Rule I

Figure 11.1 demonstrates what happens when JIT rule I is violated: The 1-2-3 pharmaceutical production process has a demand of ten units per month for each of three drugs, A, B, and C. It is clear that the demand can be met with the current resources. Occasionally, the production manager wishes to work on batches of twenty units of every product. The motivation is to save setup times, save paperwork, or because of measuring performance by quantity (a common policy constraint). The resulting process is presented in Figure 11.2, described as follows:

• At first, twenty units of product A were put into production. They went through the three-stage process: ten units were delivered to customers, and ten units were stacked in finished goods inventory.

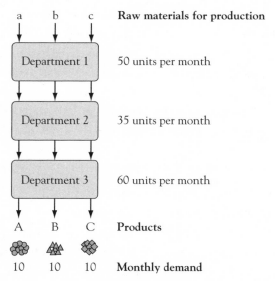

Figure 11.1. A 1-2-3 Production System with Three Products.

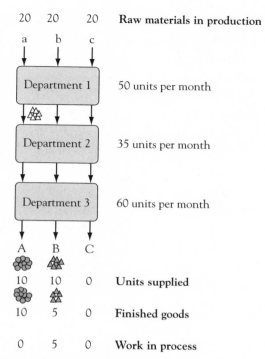

Figure 11.2. Violation of JIT Rule I.

• The twenty-unit batch of product B became stuck in department 2, and the batch was split: five units were left as WIP inventory, and fifteen units finished all three processing stages; ten of them were delivered to the customers, and five were left over in finished goods inventory.

• Units of product C were never delivered to customers.

The bottom-line result is that the company produced thirty-five units rather than thirty. However, product C was not produced at all and hence not supplied to customers. If the firm had worked by JIT rule, every product would have been produced in a quantity of ten units, and delivery to customers would have been flawless.

In a certain country, the law requires EDs to process a patient in less than four hours. To avoid breaking the law, ambulances arriving at the ED when it was full were asked to wait outside until the ED was ready to process the patient.

In an ED, a nonurgent patient is occasionally treated at the expense of an urgent one who is waiting unnecessarily.

The 40-20-40 Phenomenon

Ignoring JIT rule I creates the 40-20-40 phenomenon in organizations. This is a situation where 40 percent of the demand is supplied ahead of time, 20 percent of demand is supplied on time, and 40 percent of demand is supplied late. Observing JIT rule I "balances the line": demand that was previously delivered late will be delivered on time at the expense of the demand that was previously fulfilled too early.

In an ED, the staff can control whom they treat first, whom second, and so forth. Some patients are treated earlier than they need to be whereas treatment to others is delayed, causing adverse effects. This results from the desired sequencing of attending physician and consultant. When a consultant is on hand, prioritization should be done according to needs of the consultant.

JIT Rule II

We refer to a batch (lot) as when several units are processed sequentially one after another. We distinguish among several batch types: working (production) batches and transfer batches.

JIT Rule II: Work in small, appropriate, and smart batches.

In service or production processes, a working batch reflects several units that are processed at a work center in between two setups.

The determination of batch size is one of the important questions in planning a service or production. In the production of pharmaceuticals, if the work batches are too big, we run the risk of losing products due to expiration dates.

Batch size may vary along the process of material or information flow. For example, in a production process:

- The purchase batch for total production is 10,000 units.

- The shipment batch from the material's supplier is 1,000 units.

- Batch size when inspecting a shipment is 500 units.

- Production batch is 100 units.

- Transfer batch between workstations is 50 units.

- Batch size for delivery to customer is 250 units.

Transfer Batches

A transfer batch in health care can relate to how frequently a consultant-specialist visits the ED and at what frequency blood specimens are transferred from the ward to the laboratory. Transfer batches are a key issue in service organizations.

Transfer batch: The number of units, number of work hours, or frequency of transfer between one workstation and another.

The size of a transfer batch does not have to match the work batch (Goldratt and Fox, 1986). The transfer batch can be bigger than, smaller than, or equal to the work batch. The desire is to *make the transfer batches as small as possible*, provided this does not interfere with the process and does not cost more. Figures 11.3 and 11.4 illustrate the effects of transfer batches. Both figures have production batches of twenty-five units but different transfer batches. In the work regimen described in Figure 11.3, the twenty-five units of the batch are transferred from station 1 to station 2 once the full batch is processed in station 1. Once fully processed in station 2, the batch is transferred to station 3. After being processed in station 3, the batch is sent to the customer. The system response time under this regimen is long, t_1. In addition, there is concern that the bottleneck (station 2, for example) may have idle time when waiting for the finished batch at station 1.

In the work regimen of Figure 11.4, the production batch continues to be twenty-five units, but the transfer batch has now been cut down to five units. Once five units have been processed at a given station, they are transferred to the next workstation. The obvious result is that the response time has been dramatically reduced from t_1 to the shorter t_3. To fully exploit this improvement, we have to create willingness of the customer to accept partial shipments. Thus, the first units can be sent to the customer after a short

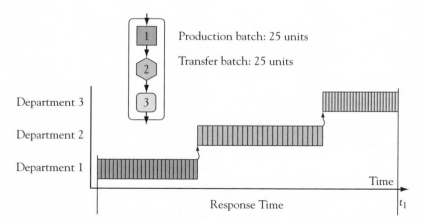

Figure 11.3. Response Time of a 1-2-3 System with a Transfer Batch of Twenty-Five Units.

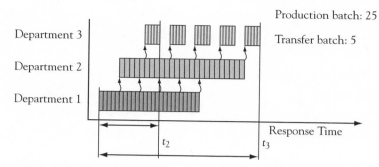

Figure 11.4. Response Time of a 1-2-3 System with a Transfer Batch of Five Units.

time period, t_2. In many situations, customers will be happy to receive some units, with the rest to follow shortly thereafter.

The ideal transfer batch is one unit. As such, every unit is transferred to the next station once it has been processed at a previous station. The reduction in response time can thus be fully exploited. The inhibitors of implementing a transfer batch of one unit include the additional conveyance needed and the added efforts in dealing with many transfers of single units from station to station. The following examples show the benefits obtained by reducing transfer batch size.

In the ED of a large hospital, some patients have their blood drawn for various tests. In the past, the staff would wait for several specimens to collect on the tray before someone would transfer them to the lab. The transfer batch was one hour (the average number of specimens in an hour), causing an average wait of half an hour for each specimen. Today, each blood specimen is transferred to the lab immediately. The resulting shorter response time of test results yields a shorter patient stay in the ED and has led to quicker diagnoses and treatment.

We should stress again that in production and maintenance processes, the transfer batch is usually measured by the number of units. In service organizations, the transfer batch is usually measured in terms of the *frequency* of transfer: one hour, two days, and so forth.

In a large logistical organization, the average response time for repairing parts lasted several months. Parts were transferred from station to station once a month. When the transfer batches were cut down to weekly batches, the response time dropped dramatically.

In a large hospital, the response time of returning lab results to the wards was reduced by a factor of 10 simply by reducing the size of the transfer batch. It turned out that the transfer batch was determined by the size of the transfer trays. Once the large trays were replaced with smaller ones, the frequency of transfers increased and response times were shortened.

The 7-Eleven chain in Tokyo is delivering goods to thousands of its stores every two hours. This enables better use of the limited and expensive shelf space of the stores.

Working (Production) Batches

A new setup is initiated only when the work on the current batch is completed and we are ready to work on the next batch.

Working batch (or *production batch*): The number of units (or labor hours) that are worked on continuously at a workstation. This is the amount of work between one setup and the next.

Let us now examine the effect of shifting from large working batches to smaller ones. We shall see what happens if we take every working batch in Figure 11.5 and split it into four working batches, as seen in Figure 11.6. Working with small working batches is a

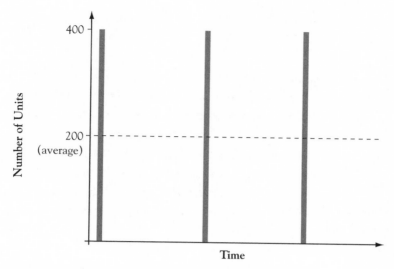

Figure 11.5. Working with Large Working Batches.

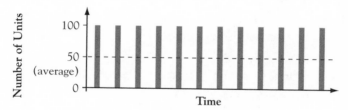

Figure 11.6. Working with Smaller Working Batches.

major contribution of Japan to the world of management. Reducing batch size results in a miraculous proportional reduction in response time and the amount of WIP. Figures 11.5 and 11.6 show that a shift from monthly batches to weekly ones reduced the amount of WIP from two hundred units to fifty units, and the system response time was probably reduced as well. The reduction of the working batch yields two positive outcomes: reduction of WIP and response times; working in small batches allows better adherence to timetables and improved quality and service to the customer.

Experience shows that the benefits from applying JIT rule II are immediate:

> In a billing department of a large hospital, preparing and mailing bills occurred once a month. The end of the month experienced peak activity, and the pressure generated problems and mistakes. To overcome this problem, the tasks were performed three times a month. The new work schedule helped overcome most billing errors and cut down the resources needed to generate and send out the bills. It also allowed better customer service to phone and mail inquiries. It substantially reduced the number of customer calls to the call center during peak hours.

> In a hospital lab, the staff used to wait for a full tray to fill up before starting the autoanalyzer. Cutting down the working batch and operating the analyzer more frequently drastically cut down the response time of returning results, which in turn resulted in better patient care. The cost of extra reagents was negligible.

> In a medical electronics firm that produced expensive imaging equipment, systems were manufactured in batches of six months' supply. While assembling the first units, engineers discovered malfunctions that required changes in the electronic boards. The firm moved to producing small batches with a two-week-supply horizon. The cycle time was drastically reduced, as was the number of rejects resulting from changes and repairs.

JIT Rule II recommends working with small, appropriate, and "smart" batches. Small batches are usually smaller than those used today. Our experience shows that in most situations, organizations work with batches that can be made smaller, resulting in reduced response times concurrent with improving other performance measures. Appropriate batches are batch sizes that are congruent with the supply rate expected by a customer. Smart batches involve using common sense in considering the special needs of the organization.

> In a hospital lab, an overall effort was made to reduce batch sizes, both for delivering specimens from wards and for running tests on autoanalyzers. One specific piece of equipment required a long setup and used expensive reagents. The operator of the machine asked permission to run larger batches as before the change. He was denied on the grounds that everybody has to adapt to the change. The new batch size was not "smart" for that specific machine.

Smart batches imply that common sense should also enter the considerations in determining batch size. The effects of reducing batch size (both working batches and transfer batches) are immediate, are relatively easy to implement, and have a major effect on reducing system response times.

Strategic Importance of Reducing Response Times and Working with Small Batches

Working with small batches allows firms to produce a large variety of products with short response times. This also enables better compatibility between products and customers and supplying them faster and at higher quality.

Working with big batches implies longer response times. This in turn requires organizations to carry larger finished goods inventory, tying down capital and increasing costs. The higher costs result from higher inventory carrying costs and the need to occasionally sell unneeded inventory at low prices.

What prevents us from working with small batches? The following factors are involved:

- Fear of increasing the number of setups
- Economies-of-scale thinking

- Fear of more complex control

- Fear of increasing cost per unit

- *Fear of increasing the number of setups.* The setup time is a non-productive time. During setup, one cannot produce or provide service. Because traditionally the setup process was long and complex, there was a tendency to avoid setups as much as possible, leading to working with large batches.

The modern approach to setups is to refrain from long and disorderly setups. Experience demonstrates that setup times can be reduced by large percentages without large investments (Shingo, 1996).

Reducing setup time by 50 percent allows a similar reduction in the working batch while maintaining the same ratio between productive time (working on the batch) and nonproductive time (setup). The result is achieving all the benefits of working with small working batches—short response time, flexible response to different customers, and better quality—without additional costs.

The framework of management by constraints shows that additional setups in resources that are not bottlenecks do not cost money. For example, Table 11.1 presents the relation between the capacity utilization and the reduction of 50 percent in the batch size in a work center with a 60 percent capacity utilization. As long as the resource is not a bottleneck, working with small batches only moderately affects the capacity utilization of this resource.

Table 11.1. Effect of Batch Size on the Load of Noncritical Resources.

Load	Large Batch	Small Batch
Percentage of productive work	50	50
Percentage of setup time	10	20
Percentage of total capacity utilization	60	70

Note: Small batch is half the size of the large batch.

• *Economies-of-scale thinking.* People are used to the concept of economies of scale where large quantities imply savings. However, economies of scale may not always be relevant and must be considered in every specific situation. When batches are processed in a system with excess capacity, economies of scale are not important. On the contrary, working with large batches increases response time and more undesirable consequences of WIP. This is a drawback, not a benefit, of economies of scale.

When a workstation is a bottleneck, setup time should be shortened as much as possible. In addition, we should check whether a specific situation would benefit by using larger batches in the bottleneck station than in other stations (Goldratt and Cox, 1992).

• *Fear of more complex control.* Working in small batches and splitting a batch into several smaller transfer batches seemingly leads to more complex control as a result of needing to control more batches. There is no doubt that shifting to smaller working and transfer batches leads to handling more batches. However, the shorter times for each batch create a situation where the number of batches in the system at any given time is *smaller* rather than bigger. Hence, follow-up and control are easier (Karp and Ronen, 1992). Moreover, working with smaller batches, along with the use of additional tools of strategic and tactical gating, complete kits, and so forth, cleans the system from congestion of work and tasks in process, so the control process becomes even simpler.

• *Increasing cost per unit.* A worker or manager who works in a system that is using the classical costing approach (see Chapter 15) for control and decision making may resist shifting to work involving smaller batches, fearing this may negatively affect the cost-per-unit measure. For example, in a station that is not a bottleneck, setup time is one hour, and the processing time of one unit is one-quarter hour, the cost per unit in a batch of one hundred is

$$T(100) = \frac{1 + (0.25 \times 100)}{100} = \frac{1 + 25}{100} = \frac{26}{100} = 0.26 \text{ hours per unit}$$

Shifting the batch size to ten will increase the cost per unit to:

$$T(10) = \frac{1 + (0.25 \times 10)}{10} = \frac{1 + 25}{10} = \frac{3.5}{10} = 0.35 \text{ hours per unit}$$

This measurement of cost per unit is a local view that causes suboptimization, especially in a workstation that is not a bottleneck. A global system view requires consideration of the total benefits versus the harms of working in large batches, which include, as mentioned earlier, the adverse effects of WIP.

JIT Rule III

Wastes are activities, processes, or use of capital that do not contribute added value to the organization, the customer, the process, or the product. The following are examples of waste:

- Overproduction
- Waiting times
- Unnecessary conveyance
- Rejected products in processing
- Surplus stock
- Poor quality
- Unnecessary space
- Capital surplus
- Overspecification and overdesign of the product or service
- Unnecessary steps and processes

JIT Rule III: Avoid wastes and activities that do not add value to the organization.

JIT Rule III is a general principle. Wastes can be dealt with through the Pareto rule, the focusing matrix, or by the principles of management by constraints.

Measurement and Control

The mere act of measuring, follow-up, and control of response times and levels of WIP bring about rapid improvement in these areas and the creation of an environment that achieves improvement. Measurement, even if not supported by other methods, results in real improvement. For more detail, see Chapter 13.

Implementing the DBR Mechanism

The DBR mechanism schedules the *controlled release* of tasks into the process, thus limiting the amount of WIP. Timing is determined by the capacity of the constraint while maintaining a buffer in front of it. Implementing DBR in systems of marketing, sales, production, development, and service leads to a significant reduction of the work process.

Quality Improvement and Reduction of the "Garbage Plant"

Poor quality in processes of sales, marketing, development, production, or service results in much rework and retreatment, thus increasing response times and the amount of WIP. Approaches for improving process quality and process control mechanisms will be presented in Chapter 17.

Avoiding Bad Multitasking

The phenomenon of bad multitasking is common in all areas of management and is especially prominent in development processes (Goldratt, 1997). This is the phenomenon of *jumping among many open tasks* that are waiting to be processed. The results of bad multitasking are a decrease in throughput, longer response times for finishing tasks, late deliveries, reduced work quality, and increased WIP, including all its drawbacks.

To demonstrate the negative effect of bad multitasking, let us analyze a situation where someone develops software modules for three projects that are managed by three different project managers. The development of each module is expected to take two weeks. The first module has to be ready in two weeks, the second in four weeks, and the third in six weeks. In reality, things happen somewhat differently, as can be seen in Figure 11.7.

The software engineer starts working on the module for project 1. At first he has a "mental" setup time: he has to immerse himself into the problem, understand it, collect the necessary data, ask questions, and arrange the work environment. After finishing this setup, he begins working on the module for project 1. After about a week, the worker bumps into the manager for project 2, who is surprised to hear that work has not yet begun on the module for her project.

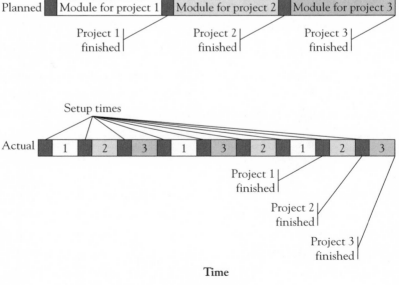

Figure 11.7. Negative Effects of Bad Multitasking.

After yielding to the pressure she applies, the developer stops working on project 1 and starts working on project 2.

First, he must start with the mental setup for project 2 and fully understand the problem well. Then he begins working on the module for project 2. The same story repeats itself after several days when he coincidentally meets the project 3 manager in the cafeteria. She, too, is surprised that her project receives low priority and that work has not yet begun on it. After pressure exerted by the manager of project 3, the developer stops working on project 2 and shifts to project 3, again having to go through a mental setup. Now project 1 manager exerts pressure because he feels his project is already late. So the developer stops working on project 3 and returns to project 1. However, he must redo the mental setup (because time passed, and he had already forgotten some things).

In the end, none of the modules was delivered on time. Furthermore, because of the additional mental setup times while switching among projects, valuable time had been lost at the bottleneck, not to mention the quality of the work.

Bad multitasking can be reduced using the following steps:

- Teach and explain.

- Apply strict control using tactical gating.

- Measure, follow up, and control the number of tasks assigned to each worker.

Field experience shows that development people occasionally work on too many tasks. We are not saying that development people should work on only one task at a time. However, two to four simultaneous open tasks are a reasonable number that will assure that the developer will not be idle when one task is held back, such as while waiting for data. A significant reduction of bad multitasking will reduce response times and increase throughput and quality.

Implementing Group Technology

Group technology is an approach where similar tasks are grouped and aggregated under specialized work groups. For example, a hospital ED may be separated into a surgical ED, internal medicine ED, pediatric ED, and gynecological ED. Within each specialized ED, the variance among patients is small, and they are more similar to each other than if there was only one general ED. Each specialized ED can thus offer more professional, structured, and uniform medical diagnosis and treatment because each employs the relevant specialists.

Group technology also exists in production processes. Work teams are assembled to be responsible for the entire product and not just one production function. Insurance companies form work teams that specialize in specific markets and defined clients.

The classical approach for operations management is to create teams that specialize functionally, where the customer or the product moves among the groups. This is demonstrated in Figure 11.8

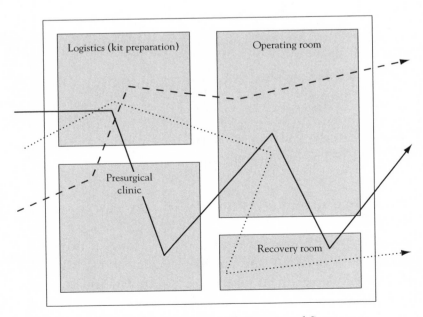

Figure 11.8. System Arrangement with Functional Structure.

for an OR situation. In the group technology approach, integrative teams provide the entire service needed by the customers in one place, as can be seen in Figure 11.9.

Figures 11.8 and 11.9 demonstrate how a complex work flow under the functional structure becomes simpler under the group technology approach. In addition, the group technology approach generates a *collective responsibility and accountability of the group* to the customer or the product. It yields faster response times, a reduction in WIP, and increased output (Burbridge, 1968). Most cases do not require added resources for achieving the improved performance.

In a claims department of a health insurance company, every customer had to go through five steps, as depicted in Figure 11.10. This was a cumbersome and annoying journey. Management decided to form three teams, each handling all five steps, as depicted in Figure 11.11. Each customer was handled by one team that performed all five tasks.

In a large governmental hospital, the ED had several subareas such as a casting room, electrocardiograph room, and so forth. Patients

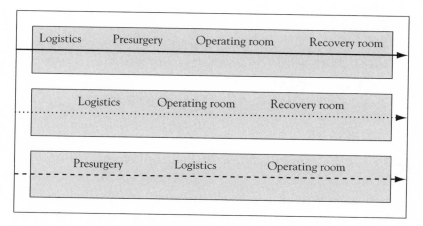

Figure 11.9. System Arrangement Using Group Technology.

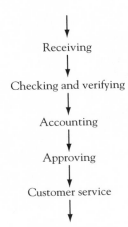

Figure 11.10. The Claims Department Before Group Technology.

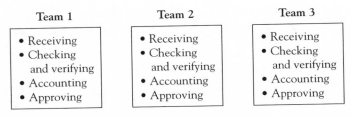

Figure 11.11. The Claims Department After Applying Group Technology.

would move from area to area according to their specific needs. Under the group technology approach, teams are brought to the patient and provide everything the patient needs in the ED.

A full (100 percent) group technology can only rarely be achieved. We cannot achieve total and full responsibility of the group for every aspect of a service or the product. There are usually some common resources shared by several groups. For example, imaging services can be common for all the specialized EDs in the example above.

Experience shows that group technology succeeds under the following conditions:

- Work volume justifies a specialized group for a long time horizon.

- The resources shared by the various teams are not bottlenecks.

- Motivation and team spirit can be created.

Working in Parallel Rather Than Serially

Performing tasks in parallel rather than serially help considerably to reduce response times. This is especially true for response times of projects, as will be discussed in detail in Chapter 20.

Chapter Summary

Reducing response times is a strategic and tactical goal for an organization. Using the approaches and techniques presented in this chapter can reduce response times severalfold.

The significant contribution of the JIT approach to management is manifested in focusing on short response times and viewing WIP as a *burden* and not as an *asset*. The JIT approach turns attention to the undesirable consequences of the WIP inventory. Other contributions of the JIT method are the techniques of using small working batches and transfer batches and shortening setup times.

Reducing response times by focusing on management by constraints, changing performance measures, using the complete kit concept, and having a global view of enhancing the firm's value significantly improves the performance of an organization.

12

The Complete Kit Concept

Objectives

- Understand the evils of incomplete kits and appreciate the value of working with complete kits

- Understand why people tend to work with incomplete kits

The complete kit concept and its theoretical background are easy to understand and not difficult to implement. This managerial tool has been implemented in various organizations with a high success rate. It is easy to adopt in every environment and situation, providing much benefit in a relatively short time. We present here the concept of a complete kit and show how it can be implemented in the health care system by demonstrating its high accomplishment rate in several medical processes in environments such as emergency departments (EDs) and operating rooms (ORs). Working with a complete kit leads to fast productivity gains. Based on our experience, it is surprising that little has been done in the medical field to use this method as an effective means to improve quality and medical services. Taking into consideration the complete kit's simplicity and effectiveness, it is somehow surprising that just-in-time (JIT) adherents like Schonberger (1986) and Suzaki (1987) pay such little attention to it. Proponents of quality management (see Chapter 17) such as Deming (1986) relate to it only implicitly by saying "do it right the first time and on time." The theory of constraints can easily be integrated into this concept. The complete kit concept is easy to adopt in the health care environment and provides much benefit in a relatively short time, as in other industries today (for example, see Coman, Koller, and Ronen, 1996; Eden and Ronen, 1993; Grosfeld-Nir and Ronen, 1998; Ronen, 1992). In this chapter, we discuss the complete kit concept and its implications for better health care management (Leshno and Ronen, 2001).

What Is a Complete Kit?

A complete kit is the readiness of the kit before the start of a procedure. There are two types: the in-kit and the out-kit. The out-kit of a given operation may be the in-kit of the next stage.

A *complete kit* in health care is the set of components and materials, medical documents, laboratory results, and other information needed to complete a given procedure, medical process, or task.

The *in-kit* of a given task is the matter and data required as an input to an operation or medical procedure.

The *out-kit* of a given task is all the material and data required as an output of an operation or medical procedure.

Drawbacks of an Incomplete Kit

To fully understand and value the complete kit concept, it is important to understand the disadvantages of working with an incomplete kit. We will demonstrate these in three areas of the health care environment: the ED, the OR, and pharmaceutical purchasing. The following represent some of the adverse consequences in trying to work without a complete kit.

More Work in Process

Any specific task in a medical environment defines a process. For the ED example, the process includes, among other things, taking the medical history of a patient, nurse and physician physical examinations, medical tests, and the conclusion reached by the physician to either discharge the patient to home or to another facility or to admit him or her to the hospital. Work in process (WIP) in the ED means, for example, people waiting for completion of the admission process. Using an incomplete kit causes more WIP, that is, more people waiting in the ED, because the specific task is invariably waiting for additional components to arrive. For example, if a specialist consultation is requested for a patient in the ED and the consultant starts the examination without having a complete kit (that is, all lab results, imaging results, and an electrocardiogram), the specialist may need another visit once the results are available. This causes more waiting time for the patient, and the consulting physician is not always available and may be considered a bottleneck. Of course, in cases of extreme emergency and danger to a patient, one can define an immediate kit of information for the given situation.

Longer Response Time

The response time is the time from the starting point of the process to its end. In the OR, the response time would be the time from when a patient is moved to the OR until he or she is moved back to the ward or to the intensive care unit. The linear (proportional) relationship between the level of WIP and the "production" response time has been widely discussed (Schonberger, 1986); more incomplete kits cause more WIP and hence a longer response time. Because the response time is considered to be a source of tactical and strategic advantage to an organization, it is extremely important to use all possible methods to reduce it to a minimum. If a patient arrives in the OR without a complete kit (for example, electrolyte data are not available), the anesthetist may decide to wait until the blood specimen has been taken and the data are available, or he or she may postpone surgery. In any case, an incomplete kit causes a longer response time.

High Variance of Quoted and Planned Response Times

It is difficult to estimate a response time when a major piece of information is missing and difficult to predict when a missing item will arrive. A longer response time means difficulties in planning and scheduling, which results in inefficient performance in the OR. When a patient arrives with a complete kit for a routine procedure or test (colonoscopy, for example), it is easy to predict the procedure response time; the response time deviation is considered relatively small. However, when a patient arrives with an incomplete kit, the response time variance increases, causing difficulties in prediction, scheduling, and planning, which in turn results in inefficient performance and poor quality of services.

Poor Quality and More Reworking

As was discussed in Chapter 10, excessive WIP causes poor-quality performance, both in level of service to a patient and in the delivery of clinical quality. Patients arriving with incomplete kits tend to wait too long in inadequate facilities. When the missing items or information arrive, they are reviewed by the physicians for the second or third time. This undoubtedly leads to poor-quality service. The clinical outcome may also be impaired, and the fact that a patient coming with an incomplete kit is doubly and even triply handled, sometimes by another physician or another shift team, causes a severe decline in quality.

Decline in Throughput

The number of patients being operated on in a specific time interval is the throughput of an OR. Using an incomplete kit in the OR results in a decline of throughput.

Decline in Productivity

Using an incomplete kit increases both setup times such as setting up the OR for the next patient and the required time per patient, taking into consideration the duplicate handling. In a paperwork environment, such as that connected with the logistics of purchasing pharmaceuticals for a health care organization, the inefficiency factor for using an incomplete kit is assessed to be approximately 80 percent (Ronen, 1992). This means that in the medical logistics systems, a process that takes 1.0 person-hours using a complete kit may be increased to 1.8 person-hours, should some materials be unavailable.

Higher Operating Expense

A high WIP causes higher operating expense due to more holding costs, more scrap, and more work put into the task. As noted by Schonberger (1986), any operation that does not add value to the process is a waste. Poor quality costs more money because more work must be performed (Deming, 1986) to complete an operation. Double setups add more expenses to the process.

Decline in Staff Motivation

Using an incomplete kit goes against the grain. It diminishes staff motivation and trust in the system when they are forced to do more and apparently unnecessary work. A prime example is that of a physician on duty in the ED needing to see many patients unnecessarily three or more times because a complete kit is not available the first time.

Increased Complexity and Control

If one works using an incomplete kit, controlling the system becomes complex and sometimes almost impossible.

Less Effort Expended to Ensure Arrival of a Missing Kit Item

Releasing an incomplete kit gives the illusion that every effort is being made to get the job done.

What Stops People from Using a Complete Kit?

If the benefits of using a complete kit are so obvious, why is it not used more often? The answer seems to center around certain obstacles on the way to assembling a complete kit.

The Efficiencies Syndrome

The "efficiencies syndrome" is the urge to have resources utilized as much as possible. Following the fallacious notion that staff should be busy all the time causes managers to have their people working on incomplete kits just so they would not be idle. More importantly, it also means more WIP, less throughput, and more operating expenses.

The basic remedy for the efficiencies syndrome is a major change in the management of the organization, such as introducing quality management (Deming, 1986), the theory of constraints, or the JIT approach, incorporating the complete kit approach into this overall concept. Indeed, a complete kit practice works best as part of a total management philosophy.

The efficiencies syndrome is counterproductive if the operation has either an internal constraint (resource bottlenecks) or an excess capacity. In the bottleneck environment, there are always other jobs that can turn into immediate throughput. In cases of excess capacity, there is pressure to use an incomplete kit just to utilize resources. There is no justification whatsoever for this because excess capacity means shorter response times. Thus, there is virtually no advantage to starting work with an incomplete kit.

Pressure for an Immediate Response

It is well known that process time is only a small part of the total response time. For example, the median response time in a large ED is about four hours whereas the actual process time is only about twenty-five minutes. Sometimes the physician starts treating a patient with an incomplete kit because of systemic pressure for immediate response, although the physician knows he or she will not be able to finish the procedure without all the necessary information.

Staff's Eagerness to Show Goodwill

As a result of management pressure, laboratory technicians, nurses, and even physicians express their goodwill by releasing incomplete kits to the medical or surgical ward. The conflict of not using a complete kit is described in the conflict-resolution diagram in Figure 12.1.

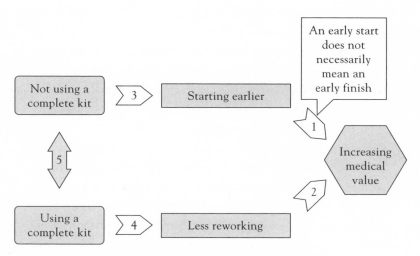

Figure 12.1. Conflict Resolution Using a Complete Kit.

The Complete Kit Concept in the Health Care System

In a paperwork environment such as that characterizing medical logistics, the rule is to start working only if the kit is complete. For example, in the purchasing of pharmaceuticals, the process will not start unless the kit includes all the documents and information needed (that is, end-user approval, budget number, and the like). In such an environment, a gatekeeper is designated as the only person authorized to release jobs. Clearly, the task cannot be finished if a document or a form is missing. The main point is not to start until all the documents are at hand.

> Colonoscopy is one of the most significant diagnostic and therapeutic applications of endoscopy because it can diagnose potentially curable colonic cancers that would be missed by other techniques, and it can be used for the removal of potentially precancerous adenomatous polyps. Most initial colonoscopies are performed in a gastroenterology department to investigate findings on an abnormal barium enema study or to elucidate the cause of gastrointestinal bleeding. The ability to examine the whole colon is also useful in the treatment of some patients with inflammatory bowel disease and in those with a family history of colonic polyps or cancer. The complete kit of a colonoscopy includes various medical technologies that are needed for the procedure, such as the endoscope, various medications, a resuscitation cart ready for any medical life support situation, and so forth. An important procedure before initiating a colonoscopy is the preparation of the patient with laxatives and tap-water enemas or by a total-gut lavage with a nonabsorbable electrolyte solution. At least twenty-four hours are needed to achieve good preparation. If a patient cancels a colonoscopy scheduled for the next day, another patient on the list is scheduled instead. However, the new patient arrives at the clinic unprepared, and the result in many cases is an incomplete examination and

the need for a second colonoscopy. The damage is twofold: there is wasted medical resources, and the patient does not receive good health care. Moreover, the results of the colonoscopy may be inconclusive, and there may be a misdiagnosis. Had the gastroenterology department worked with a complete kit, situations like these would be rare. Therefore, it is important to instruct the staff not to schedule patients for colonoscopy who have not undergone full preparation. It is preferable to absorb the waste of time and resources due to cancellation rather than to enter a procedure without a complete kit.

Other methods can be used to improve the operation of the department. For example, if the cancellation rate is 10 percent, one should overbook for colonoscopy 10 percent above the capacity of the department and then, three days before the scheduled date, call everyone to confirm their arrival. Using the complete kit method will increase the production and the clinical quality of the department by at least 30 percent.

One of the authors of this book was scheduled for hernia surgery. On checking into the hospital, he was asked what medications, if any, he is taking. He responded that he is taking only vitamins and low-dose aspirin. The admitting nurse surprisingly asked if he had been instructed to stop taking aspirin ten days before surgery. He had not been instructed to do so; the admission was cancelled and surgery postponed. As a result, there was an empty bed in the ward, there was a vacant slot in the OR schedule, and valuable resources were wasted. The incomplete instructions given to the patient are an example of an incomplete kit and its adverse effects.

As demonstrated in the next subsections, implementation of the complete kit concept in a health care environment is well supported by modern management philosophies and techniques such as the theory of constraints, quality management (see Chapter 17), and the JIT approach.

Theory of Constraints Support

According to the theory of constraints, the goal of a health care organization is to provide good-quality medical services in the present as well as in the future. Using the complete kit paradigm will increase the number of patients receiving appropriate medical treatment, increasing their satisfaction and the quality of their treatment. In the theory of constraints terminology, working with an incomplete kit is considered a "policy constraint" and should therefore be eliminated.

Quality Management Support

An organization that works according to the quality management principles will soon come around to adopting the complete kit concept. Along the route to improving processes, many negative effects (like high WIP, misdiagnosed patients, and so forth) will be traced to the use of incomplete kits. Quality management tools—control charts, the Pareto diagram, and others—can maintain and monitor the complete kit process. The quality management control cycle will support avoidance of incomplete kits. A control chart of the process response time will detect the exceptional batches. A cause-and-effect diagram will get at the root of the problem: an incomplete kit. A Pareto diagram can show the main contributors to the phenomenon (classification by either customers or the missing items). Reduction of response time, monitored by the appropriate control chart, will show the improvement.

Implementing the Complete Kit in a Health Care Organization

The following steps are suggested to implement a complete kit process:

1. The introduction of a complete kit process has to be part of a major change in the organization. It has to be part of a JIT approach, quality management, or theory of constraints implementation.

2. Top management has to be involved in the process. Without the support of top management, there will be tremendous pressure from second-tier managers to start processing incomplete kits in the belief that this will speed up the work.

3. One person has to be appointed in each department to take charge. Usually it is the gatekeeper ("gater"), that is, the person who releases the jobs or patients to the process. This should be part of tactical gating.

4. The process must be monitored: Pareto charts need to be drawn, classifying incomplete kits by types of treatments, types of patients, or by the missing components. Using cause-and-effect techniques (fishbone diagrams, effect-cause-effect, and the like), causes are sought and corrective actions applied. The usual quality management way of improving processes may be employed here with good effects.

5. Employees and internal customers need to be informed of the change. Several organizations that have adopted the concept have designed special workshops to cope with this issue. The use of personal computer simulations and demonstrations using special software has been introduced into the educational process.

6. External customers (such as health maintenance organizations [HMOs]) should be notified that they will get better due-date performance and better quoted response times if they submit a complete kit. For example, HMOs should be informed that the laboratories are using the complete kit method and, hence, will expect that all patients referred will arrive with a compete kit.

7. The term "complete kit" should be redefined from time to time according to the circumstances. A good rule is: work smart and beware of inertia.

8. Components and materials should be ordered in complete kits. Instead of ordering batches of the same components, the provider should order a kit from his or her supplier. This applies to both internal and external suppliers.

9. All activities should be synchronized, ensuring that the out-kit of the current activity is the in-kit of the next one.

10. Components and procedures need to be standardized whenever possible. The more standard items, the more likely it is that a complete kit will soon be available.

Implications for Health Care Management Information Systems

The management information system (MIS) department in a health care organization has to support activities with certain tools to enable a complete kit. Thus, a kit management procedure should be developed. For any activity, the MIS department should supply the relevant documents and information to give a compete kit and ensure that the activity does not proceed until the kit is complete.

Insofar as most of the items in a medical kit are medical information and data, an MIS plays a major role in reinforcing and implementing the complete kit paradigm and should be designed accordingly. Using an intranet (or other communication tools), the MIS can maintain the complete kit framework by using an automatic checklist and providing users the missing items for a complete kit. In cases where a health care organization has a data warehouse, it can deliver the information items needed automatically. An intranet system can also search for missing items. If some of the items in the kit are created outside the organization, "smart agents" using the Internet and other communication facilities can be used to automatically deliver missing items to the kit. Electronic data interchange, networked computing, the Internet, intranet, extranet, and data warehouse (for example, Hölzer and others, 1999) can contribute to better completion of the kit. For example, a computer-aided system using the complete kit concept can reduce the time for approval of a new drug by the Food and Drug Administration (FDA). The complete kit application in this case would involve collecting many items automatically by scanning data into a computer, providing indexed data online for quick retrieval, running an automatic checklist, and once the kit is complete, sending the data on a CD-ROM to the FDA.

Information systems that support the complete kit concept can be part of enterprise resource planning or special-purpose systems, like those described by Czuchry, Yasin, and Norris (2000).

Implications for Medical Purchasing and Logistics Departments

The purchasing department would be required to change its procedures as follows according to the complete kit concept:

- It would purchase complete kits. The orders would be in kits rather than in components.
- This would force the purchasing department to work with fewer suppliers and purchase more items from each supplier.
- Suppliers would be evaluated not only by price, response time, and quality but also by the completeness of the kits.

Field Results

A study of health care organizations and industrial organizations that have implemented the complete kit concept show that it has reduced WIP and cut response time by a factor of three. In one implementation in a health care system, using a complete kit together with small batches and drum-buffer-rope scheduling, as well as tactical gating, led to a substantial increase (up to dozens of percentage points) of throughput.

Although it is too early to make any comprehensive assessment of the value of introducing the complete kit concept in health care organizations, preliminary results show a major improvement in the following areas of health care: EDs, ORs, outpatient clinics, and radiology departments.

Chapter Summary

The complete kit is a well-established concept, tried and trusted in manufacturing, with considerable potential for improving health care systems. It can be used to gain a strategic competitive edge because of the faster response times, lower prices, and better quality that it yields.

Our experience shows that the health care system is an environment in which the complete kit concept can be applied with good effects. Experience in training and educating executives, managers, physicians, nurses, and other paramedical staff shows that in many cases the practitioners need a formal framework, even though their intuition about the complete kit is good. They need a theoretical background and methodological framework such as those presented in this chapter to better cope with the pressure from supervisors to work with an incomplete kit. Today's medical staff does not have the managerial backing to say no to an incomplete kit. The intention of this chapter is to impress the management of health care settings to provide such backing.

13

Performance Measures and Managerial Control

- Understand the need to evaluate performance and to measure it

- Learn how to use the six global performance measures in practice

Global Performance Measures

As we have seen in previous chapters, local performance measures may distort the decision-making process and lead to suboptimization. A measure such as cost per unit may result in the production of large batches, which leads to excess inventory and due date delays. A measure such as the number of police tickets will not achieve the goal of reducing the number of traffic accidents and smoothing traffic flow. A measure of the number of patients seen in an emergency department (ED) may lead to early discharge and suboptimal treatment. Thus, we need global performance measures that will yield the benefits described below.

Voicing Management Policy Regarding an Organization's Goals

People behave according to how they are measured: "Tell me how you behave, and I'll tell you how you are measured." Clear and simple measures will broadcast management policy in an unambiguous way. Improving these measures should improve the value of a firm in a business environment and advance organizational goals in a not-for-profit environment.

Aid Decision Making

It is easier for top management to consider different alternatives vis-à-vis the organizational goal so that the chosen alternative will enhance the firm's value for its shareholders. However, middle management will frequently find it difficult to see the direct link between action in the field and enhancing the firm's value. Thus, we need performance measures that translate the organizational goal into operative language.

The performance measures are thus an intermediary between decision makers and organizational goals. For example, in managing the introduction of a new drug, time to market is an important measure for value enhancement. The project manager will seek to reduce the time to market.

Control

Performance measure can be used by middle management as a tool for routine control. When measurement reveals problems, it enables correcting them. When it reveals improved performance, it enables learning from successes and replicating them elsewhere in the organization. Performance measures enable an organization to monitor whether the organization is moving toward achieving its goals in the short and long term and what corrective actions are needed to improve performance.

Reward and Evaluation

Good performance measures can serve as part of a system of evaluation and reward in an organization to improve worker motivation and advance organizational goals.

Ability to Decentralize

A CEO, talented as can be, cannot centralize all decisions within an organization. Appropriate performance measures, by which the CEO and his or her subordinates are measured, allow decentralized decision-making processes. Appropriate performance measures should have the following characteristics:

- *Global and effective:* Effective measures are such that their improvement in business organizations significantly advances the achievement of the organizational goal and enhances the firm's value, and in not-for-profit organizations, they advance organizational goals.
- *Simple and clear:* "What will not be simple, simply will not be." Measures should be clear, simple, and easily measured.
- *Based on the satisficer approach:* Measures should be satisfactory and not necessarily perfect or optimal. Implementing performance measures in an organization is not simple, and therefore, it is advisable to proceed gradually. The desire to implement a set of accurate and perfect measures may prove too difficult and lead to abandoning the process.
- *Founded on easy and simple data collection:* It is desirable to use data from existing databases in the organization and have the users of the measures be the ones collecting the data.
- *Customized to the organization:* The attempt to adopt "as is" measures that have succeeded elsewhere may end in disappointment. The organization must gradually build its own appropriate measures or properly adapt others.

The Six Global Performance Measures

We present a general set of six generic performance measures that can be expanded or reduced according to every organization's needs. The first three measures were defined by Goldratt and Cox (1992) and the others by Eden and Ronen (1993). The global performance measures represent output measures, input measures, and process measures, as follows:

- Throughput (T)

- Operating expenses (OE)

- Inventory (I)

- Response time (RT)

- Quality (Q)

- Due date performance (DDP)

Throughput

Throughput is the effective output of an organization.

> The throughput of traffic police is reducing the number of accidents and improving traffic flow. It is not the number of tickets issued.

> A hospital operating room (OR) should be interested in the income from procedures and surgeries, not hours of operation. The focus should be on output, not input. Throughput is the monetary contribution of the procedures.

———————

In business organizations, throughput is defined as the *cash flow* generated from sales—more specifically: total *actual sales* minus *real variable costs* of those sales.
Actual sales: Sales that were actually carried out, minus returns and cancelled sales.
Real variable costs: Raw materials, components, subcontractors, commissions, and so forth.

———————

A company is committed to deliver every month 100 units of product A, 100 units of product B, and 100 units of product C at a selling price of $10 per unit. The company has no work-in-process inventory, and there is no finished goods inventory at the beginning of the month. The real variable costs for each unit are $4. The company decides to produce 200 units of A, 150 units of B, and no units of product C. This is a seemingly strange decision. If there are well-defined demands, why not produce accordingly? In reality, firms frequently do not produce according to market demands and justify their actions on grounds of "economies of scale," reducing per unit cost, savings in additional administrative work, or savings on additional machine setups. Sometimes a measure is the number of units produced, with no regard to market demand, which results in inappropriate production decisions. The throughput of the above system, using the data in Table 13.1, is calculated as follows, with T representing throughput:

$$T = 100 \, (10 - 4) + 100 \, (10 - 4) + 0 =$$
$$100(6) + 100(6) + 0 = 600 + 600 + 0 = \$1,200$$

The output from products A and B is calculated based on 100 units that were actually sold (the surplus units will be counted in the inventory measure). In our example, production is 350 units (compared with a demand of 300), but the throughput is only $1,200, less than the potential throughput of $1,800 (if the plant would have produced and sold what the market demands).

Table 13.1. Calculation of Throughput.

	Product A	Product B	Product C
Demand (units)	100	100	100
Selling price per unit ($)	10	10	10
Real variable costs per unit ($)	4	4	4
Actual production (units)	200	150	0

It should be noted that in many places, middle management is occasionally measured by the number of units produced; this is occasionally the "organizational language." Such organizations still talk about units sold, tons, and so forth. In the insurance industry, the measure of production (total new premiums sold in a period) is still thriving. This may lead to accepting orders that will result in losses.

Measuring throughput in monetary units (dollars) sends a message throughout the organization that "we mean business" and helps meet due-date performance vis-à-vis customers by focusing everybody on creating effective output. In one organization, we encountered a department manager who successfully implemented the philosophy and refused to produce surplus, saying "This will not give throughput to the firm." This reflects a successful implementation of measures that become part of the organizational language.

> Both public and business-oriented hospitals have large fixed costs, mainly for personnel. The variable costs are only 10 to 15 percent of the budget. We should focus on throughput as the generator of contribution.

Operating Expenses

Operating expenses include direct labor, indirect labor, and rent and other fixed expenses. Another definition of operating expenses are the fixed costs for converting inventory into throughput (Goldratt and Cox, 1992). These expenses are fixed expenses of the organization in the short term and the medium term. Fluctuations in demand only marginally affect the direct labor costs. The operating-expense approach requires looking at the whole organization and evaluating whether expenses increased or decreased. The manager should evaluate any suggestion for change or improvement to determine if operating expenses will increase or decrease and the effect on throughput.

> A large enterprise hired the services of a consulting firm. After analyzing some data and comparing the enterprise with similar ones in the market, the consultants advised a cutback of 10 percent in the costs

of indirect labor. The CEO summoned the division managers and instructed them to cut 10 percent of indirect labor costs. This was immediately implemented despite the tense labor relations between the workers' union and management. How was this achieved? Simply, some of the indirect workers were reclassified as direct labor. Obviously, operating expenses did not decrease, and no savings were achieved.

Inventory

Inventory is classified into three categories that require different treatment: raw materials inventory, work-in-process (WIP) inventory, and finished goods inventory. The value of the three inventory types will be measured in the cost of *raw materials only*. Hence, the value of WIP inventory will not include any additional components reflecting the work invested, and the same is true for the finished goods inventory. The reason for measuring all inventories in terms of raw materials is that all conversion costs are considered fixed operating expenses. This creates convenience and transparency in calculating and analyzing inventories. For example, an increase in the WIP inventory is obviously not from a change in the way various costs have been loaded but, rather, from a real increase in quantities. This allows for quick corrective actions.

Note that this measurement method is different from the way the WIP inventory is measured in financial accounting. The accounting measures gradually increase the value of WIP inventory according to the labor hours invested in it.

In health care organizations, the WIP inventory reflects patients in the system, whether waiting or being cared for. WIP is extremely important and, therefore, must be measured. Patients waiting to enter the system (for example, patients on a waiting list for organ transplantation) represent the raw materials inventory.

Response Time

Response time is a general term for various time measures that include lead time, cycle time, time-to-market, and response time. For more accurate definitions, see Cox and Blackstone (1998) and Cox and Spencer (1998). We simply relate to system response times by one term, "response time." The organization must identify its main processes and measure their response times.

An appropriate measure of response times is one that looks at the process from the perspective of the customer. The measurement should include the actual response times, without special allowances for the responsibility of someone else. For example, patients are concerned with the total time they spend in the system, including various waits. They do not care who is responsible for a longer-than-usual wait.

Quality

Measures of quality contribute to organizational enhancement. Every organization must define its relevant quality measures, for example:

- Percentage of products or services achieved correctly the first time

- Costs of "nonquality" (size of the "garbage plant")

- Customer satisfaction

- Percentage of rehospitalizations within two days after discharge

- Number of customer complaints

In health care organizations, we focus on two types of quality issues: service quality and clinical quality

Due Date Performance

Due date performance reflects an organization's reliability in meeting deadlines. This measure, especially the last two bulleted items below, is usually not relevant for health care organizations but is presented here for the sake of completeness. Due date performance can be measured in several ways:

• *Percentage of on-time performance:* Measuring the percentage of products, services, or milestones that were completed on time. Even though this is a simple measure, in situations with wide variation in the value of services or products, this measure can distort reality by encouraging the production of the "cheap-and-easy" products. In such cases, the products should be classified into families, and due date performance should be measured for each family separately.

Occasionally organizations set a standard for providing a service or delivery—quoted response time—and one should measure adherence to this standard.

• *Delayed revenue collection as a result of not being on time (back orders):* This measure calculates at the end of every period the amount of money of orders not yet delivered. For example, order X, valued at $200,000 has not yet been delivered, as well as order Y, valued at $100,000. The total value of nonreceived payments due to back orders is, therefore, $300,000. This measure is simple, useful, understandable, and easy to monitor, and it takes into account the length of the delays.

• *Dollar days.* This method calculates the due date performance as the sum of the cash value of orders multiplied by the number of days of delay.

Table 13.2 presents an example of three delayed orders. The dollar-days measure is calculated for June 1. This better reflects the

Table 13.2. Due Date Performance Using the Dollar-Days Measure.

Order Number	Order Value ($ thousands)	Delivery Date	Days Late	Dollar Days for June 1 (millions)
351	100	January 1	150	15
352	200	February 1	120	24
353	300	March 1	90	27
Total dollar days for delayed orders				66

economic value of the delays but is not intuitively appealing to managers and workers and is rarely used. We recommend that organizations try to first use the back-orders measure of the previous section and only then move to the dollar-days measure.

Calculating Profit

We can conceptually define the profit of a firm using the above-presented measures as follows:

Profit (P) = Throughput (T) – Operating Expenses (OE)

The importance of this relation is that it forces decision makers in an organization to think globally. Saving two labor hours in some activity or seven minutes of service time is not necessarily relevant. The important issues are the effect of decisions on global performance measures—the throughput or operating expenses—and, as a result, on profit. Therefore, in organizational decision-making processes, the following questions must be asked:

- Will organizational output increase as a result of the decision?

- Will the operating expenses decrease as a result of the decision?

- Will the decision increase the difference of throughput minus operating expenses?

Long-term decision making must also take into account the effect of decisions on investments and tax issues.

Adapting Global Performance Measures to an OR

A system of performance measures must be adapted for every organization. Let us consider the case of an OR in a hospital. We will first relate to the six global measures:

- *Throughput:* The number of operations by patient mix or operation type. In a for-profit hospital, the throughput of the OR can be measured by monetary contributions (revenues for surgery minus real variable costs).

- *Operating expenses:* Rent for the OR and payment for surgeons, anesthetists, nurses, and administrative and cleaning staff. On the other hand, the costs associated with temporary seasonal workers or workers of a subcontractor who do not work on a regular basis (where the number of workers can be changed in response to workload) are considered real variable costs.

- *Inventory:* Number of patients waiting in the OR itself and number waiting in the preparation room.

- *Response time:* Time from summoning a patient from the ward to the end of surgery or time from when a patient enters the OR until leaving for the recovery room. In situations where the surgeon, anesthetist, or the OR itself is the bottleneck, it is recommended to measure the time from the end of finishing with one patient until the first incision on the next patient.

- *Quality:* Two measures: clinical quality and service quality.

- *Due date performance:* meeting the OR schedule.

The six global measures form a good starting basis. As appropriate, we may delete some of them, add others, or both. In the OR example, we can drop the nonrelevant measure of due date performance and replace it with, for example, two other measures:

1. Percentage of patients rejected for surgery

2. Percentage of patients arriving in the OR with an incomplete kit

Note that in not-for-profit organizations, there is a tendency to perform extensive and seemingly endless research on finding appropriate performance measures. They should adopt a satisficer approach. First, start with two to three acceptable, yet not ideal, measures so that measuring can begin right away. Then, as time goes by, measures can be refined and others added. There is no sense in delaying measurement until the "perfect" measure is found. The lost time translates into inferior performance.

> There are not many agreed-on measures for clinical quality in an ED. We can start immediately by using such measures as the percentage of patients returning to the ED, the percentage of patients who spend more than six hours in the ED, or both.

The Measurements Profile and Global Decision Making

The measurements profile is a tool for aiding in global decision making. The tool examines alternative decisions using the organizational global performance measures. The use of the measurements profile examines the alternatives by the six global measures presented earlier. This is a two-dimensional matrix whose columns present the different alternatives, and the rows present the performance of the measures, as outlined in Table 13.3. The measurements profile presents a succinct picture of each alternative and thus enables an easier comparison of the effect of each alternative on the various dimensions of organizational performance. A use of this profile across an organization contributes to the decision-making

Table 13.3. The Measurements Profile.

Performance Measure	Alternative A	Alternative B
Throughput (T)		
Operating expenses (OE)		
Inventory (I)		
Response time (RT)		
Quality (Q)		
Due date performance (DDP)		

process by having everyone speak the same common and under-standable language.

The above six global measures are not the only measures useful for decision making. As seen by the OR example, some of the six measures can be deleted (if not relevant) and others added, if needed. In the following chapters, we present some uses of the measurements profile in various decision-making problems.

Chapter Summary

Performance measures are a control tool for guiding and navigating managers in an organization. In many situations, an appropriate change of performance measures can bring about fast and signifi-cant improvement in organizational performance and enhancing organizational value. The global performance measures presented in this chapter help organizations focus on activities that improve performance and thus better achieve their goals.

14

Effects of Fluctuations, Variability, and Uncertainty on the System

Objectives

- Understand why variability is one of the biggest enemies of health care systems and why we need to manage it

- Understand why traditional approaches to managing variability have failed and how new approaches can better manage it

Fluctuations

The uncertainty related to malfunctions, faults, and disruptions is referred to as "fluctuations." This serves as a general term for all the seemingly unexpected situations of problems, malfunctions, interruptions, and disturbances.

Murphy's Law says that if something can go wrong, it will, and it will cause the maximal damage at the most inconvenient time. The law is occasionally phrased as the "bread-and-butter law." If a buttered slice of bread can drop to the floor, it will; if it drops, it will fall buttered side down.

Some would add that if the slice falls buttered side up, we had spread the butter on the wrong side.

The O'*Toole principle* adds that "Murphy was an optimist."

Sources of Fluctuations

Fluctuations can be classified by their source:

1. Fluctuations in demand
   - Seasonality
   - Technological changes and changes in preferences
2. Fluctuations in capacity
   - Variation of work rate at different stations
   - Variation in setup times, both physical and mental ones
   - Malfunctions: machine failure, computer crash, and the like
   - Employee absenteeism
   - Scheduling and timing problems
   - Incomplete kits
3. Fluctuations in quality
   - Unexpected defects
4. Fluctuations in the availability of materials and parts
   - Problems with quality of materials and components
   - Delays in supply
   - Supply problems (less than ordered, different from what was ordered, and so forth)

Fluctuations occur in the emergency department (ED) of a hospital due to the following:

- Uncertainty in the diagnosis

- Unavailability of consultant-specialists

- Unavailability of operating rooms

- Unavailability of critical resources

- Uncertainty of demand

Evolution of Fluctuations in a Process

Consider the planning of a new line of services, products, or development, depicted in Figure 14.1. Every task that enters the system (a patient receiving treatment, a request to develop a "smart" patient record, or assembly in production) must go through stations 1, 2, and 3. Let us assume that $15 million has been targeted for creating this process. The developers are faced with three alternatives for buying equipment, each costing $15 million. Figures 14.2, 14.3, and 14.4 present each alternative using a cost-utilization (CUT)

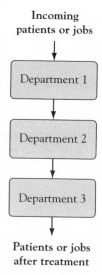

Figure 14.1. The Planned Process.

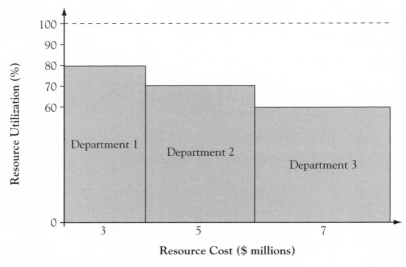

Figure 14.2. A CUT Diagram for Alternative A.

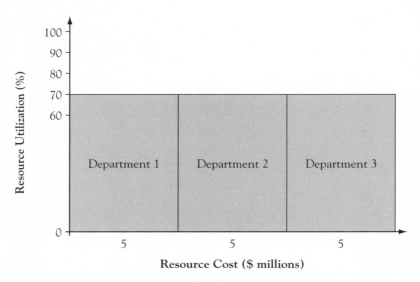

Figure 14.3. A CUT Diagram for Alternative B.

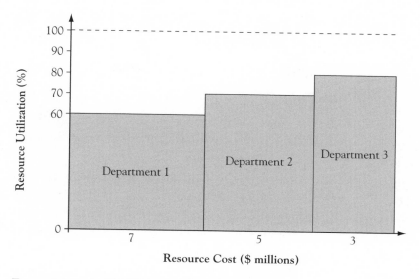

Figure 14.4. A CUT Diagram for Alternative C.

diagram. The CUT diagram presents, as we have seen before, the *average* utilization of the resources.

Which Alternative Is Best for the Organization?

Seemingly all three alternatives provide a reasonable solution. All seem to have excess capacity. However, the CUT diagram presents only the average utilization of the resources. In reality, utilization is not constant and varies due to fluctuations. Hence, considering only average utilization can lead to poor decisions.

There are two types of fluctuations: internal fluctuations and cumulative fluctuations.

Internal Fluctuations

Internal fluctuations come from the station itself and affect its performance. Internal fluctuation can result, for example, from a computer crash at a station, idling the station for a while and increasing the work rate the rest of the time. Other sources of fluctuations can be worker absenteeism, quality problems, and having a good day with above-average achievements.

Cumulative Fluctuations

The cumulative fluctuations result from performance in preceding stages of the process. Consider, for example, a group of hikers marching in a single file. Where would you rather be, at the head of the line or at the end of the line? The average speed at the head of the line is seemingly the same as that at the end of the line. However, experience shows that those at the end will occasionally have to run to keep up and occasionally halt as a result of the cumulative fluctuations of all the hikers ahead of them. The standard deviation of the speed of a walker at the end of the line is bigger than at the beginning of the line. This is described in more detail by Goldratt and Cox (1992). The behavior of fluctuations in the line is similar: the farther a resource is from the beginning of the process, the higher the cumulative fluctuations.

Let us now examine the CUT diagrams of the three alternatives where the diagrams present both the average and the variance of the capacity resulting from the internal fluctuations of the stations and the cumulative fluctuations of the preceding stations (Figures 14.5, 14.6, and 14.7). Looking at the information presented in these figures, it is clear that alternative A is the preferred choice because even at peak utilization, there is no bottleneck despite the cumulative fluctuations. With alternative B, there is almost a bottleneck part of the time, and this should be treated as if there is an actual bottleneck during these times.

The cumulative fluctuations create, some of the time, a bottleneck at department 3 of alternative C. This situation is typical for activities of testing, evaluation or calibration, or other departments at the end of the process. Because of delays in earlier stations, such departments are underutilized most of the time. However, when a "wave" of work arrives, there is a shortage of resources, and the station becomes the process bottleneck. Even though on the average

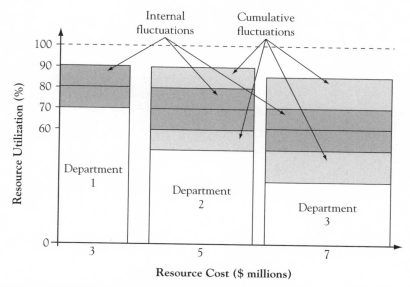

Figure 14.5. Alternative A with Internal and Cumulative Fluctuations.

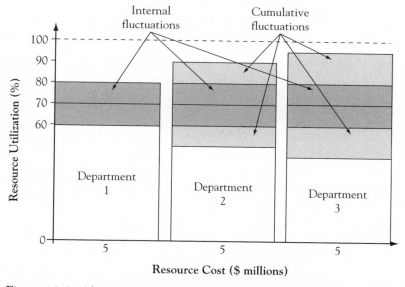

Figure 14.6. Alternative B with Internal and Cumulative Fluctuations.

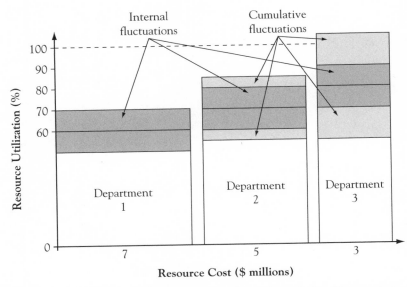

Figure 14.7. Alternative C with Internal and Cumulative Fluctuations.

such departments have adequate capacity, they become a bottleneck most of the time. The following sections of this chapter present ways to overcome this situation. We also present other ways to protect against cumulative fluctuations, such as building a buffer in front of department 3, which is the system bottleneck.

Elements of Capacity

The maximal (theoretical) capacity can be broken down into three parts (see also Cox and Spencer, 1998):

- Nominal capacity of the resource

- Protective capacity of the resource

- Excess capacity of the resource

The *nominal* capacity of the resource is the average capacity utilized for performing its tasks. The *protective* capacity of the resource is that part of the capacity that is targeted to overcome the internal and cumulative fluctuations in the load of the resource. These fluctuations result from changing demand, availability of personnel, availability of raw materials, malfunctions, and so forth. This capacity protects the system against routine fluctuations. It is not intended to protect against large and unexpected fluctuations that are rather rare, such as hurricanes, ongoing strikes, and the like.

The system bottlenecks are expensive or scarce resources; thus, the system has difficulty in creating a protective capacity for them. However, systems must create protective capacity in noncritical resources. This will assure that the bottlenecks will not be idle because of delays of work flow in the noncritical resources.

The *excess capacity* of the resource is that part of the maximal capacity of the resource that is not used, not during routine operations and not during increased utilization as a result of fluctuations.

Several conclusions emanate from this analysis:

1. During the planning stage for services, products, or development, it is not enough to consider the nominal capacity. Planning according to averages can be compared with the situation of the statistics professor who drowned in a lake with an average depth of twelve inches.

   Demand should be sorted by seasonality. For example, in an ED, there is an obvious difference between the pressure during the day and during the night. A system analysis should consider two separate EDs, a day ED and a night ED.

2. In situations of large fluctuations during peak times, the system must be planned to meet the peaks and to find ways to "sell the excess capacity" during off-peak times. For example, a restaurant whose primary business is during evening hours can try to increase sales during lunch by offering "business lunch" menus.

3. A system needs protective capacity. On a local level, this can be viewed as excess and waste. However, from a global

perspective, the protective capacity protects the throughput of the bottlenecks and assures achieving maximal output for the whole system.

4. Resources with a capacity utilization exceeding 85 percent are considered bottlenecks and must be managed accordingly.

5. While planning a service or production, we need to arrange sufficient protective capacity. The Japanese, for example, tend to build service and production systems with an average utilization of 70 percent.

6. The concept of "line balancing" is not consistent with reality, which has fluctuations in the system. Experience shows that a service or product line consists of resources with differing costs, some being scarce or expensive. We should maintain adequate protective capacity for the cheap resources so that they can operate continually and allow focusing on bottlenecks.

Traditional Approaches to Managing Fluctuations and Uncertainty

Traditional management employs a variety of approaches to face different types of fluctuations:

Traditional Approaches to Managing Fluctuations in Demand

- *Finished goods inventory:* Traditional management solves the problems of demand fluctuations by carrying a large finished goods inventory, occasionally along with many warehouses in proximity to customers. This is usually an expensive solution.

- *Special sales:* When there is a decline in sales or with the accumulation of a large inventory, special discounts are offered. The sales personnel focus on selling what they have on hand as opposed to selling what the market demands.

Traditional Approaches to Managing Capacity Fluctuations

- *High levels of work-in-process (WIP) inventory:* To overcome capacity fluctuations and concurrently meet market requirements for quick response, an organization builds up high levels of WIP inventory. This is to assure that bottlenecks do not become idle due to insufficient work flow from preceding stations or due to the lack of available materials or parts. The evils of excessive inventories are obvious.

- *Buying excess capacity:* It is not uncommon to see organizations create a big and expensive excess capacity to meet demand fluctuations.

- *Expediting:* Expediting orders can solve local problems for some customers but introduces tension into the system and diminishes economic output.

- *Automation and full computerization of the organization:* Automation or complex computerization is sometimes used as a (rather expensive) solution to overcome market fluctuations. However, without a change in processes and work procedures, the organization may carry on as before, reaching the same undesirable consequences faster and more orderly.

Traditional Approaches to Managing Fluctuations in Quality

- *Overproduction (spares):* Lack of control and an abundance of rejections frequently push managers to overproduction, thus protecting against an unexpected high number of rejects.

- *Repairs:* Creation of repair teams and repair stations is intended to solve problems of failure and rejects.

- *Final inspection and product sorting:* With this approach to quality management (see Chapter 17), at the end of each process one establishes a sorting station to sort good-quality products from poor-quality ones. This is a wasteful approach that does not prevent continued production or development of inferior products. Even so, in many instances, software-developing companies establish labor-intensive testing departments.

Traditional Approaches to Manage Fluctuations in Availability or Materials and Parts

- *Raw materials and parts inventory:* Many organizations carry high levels of raw materials and components inventory to overcome situations of delays in supply and delivery.

- *Inspection for incoming materials and components:* In situations where a customer cannot depend on the quality of work of suppliers, there is a need to establish a testing center to sort and screen the incoming shipments.

The approaches of traditional management are usually based on responses to fluctuations that have already happened or to ones associated with expensive investment in resources.

The Focused Management Approach to Managing Fluctuations in the Health Care System

Fluctuations must be managed and not responded to when they happen, in an *effective* manner on the one hand and with *minimal costs* on the other. We distinguish between two ways of managing and dealing with fluctuations: protecting against fluctuations and reducing fluctuations.

Protecting Against Fluctuations

Creating protective capacity is just one of several methods to protect against fluctuations. There are various approaches:

- *Building a buffer ahead of the bottleneck.* Building a buffer and managing it using the drum-buffer-rope (DBR) approach is a simple and effective way to reduce fluctuations. The uniqueness of this approach is the building of one buffer and not spreading the WIP across the entire system. This brings about quick results in terms of increasing output and reducing response times.
- *Creating protective capacity or excess capacity.* Creating this protection is immediate. Excess capacity can be achieved through the purchase of resources or through agreement with subcontractors. This is a relatively expensive approach.
- *Building a buffer of finished goods inventory.* In situations of a market constraint when customers request fast response times, one must build a buffer of finished goods that will cushion the demand fluctuations.
- *Building an overflow buffer after the bottleneck.* In industrial plants, one should arrange storage space and storage facilities after the bottleneck. This will allow the bottleneck to keep working when there are delays in stations that follow it.
- *Building a buffer of raw materials and parts.* Building a buffer of raw materials and parts protects the system against the possible fluctuations in their supply.

Protecting against fluctuations by creating excess capacity, protective capacity, or the right buffers in the right places can be done rather quickly. The effect of these protective measures, specifically the right buffers and the DBR mechanism, is immediate and yields short-term results. The problem is that this improvement, as big as it may be, is a one-time achievement. After the initial results, further improvement in protective methods against fluctuations is slow and lengthy and must be accompanied by activities to reduce fluctuations.

Reducing Fluctuations

There are several mechanisms to reduce fluctuations. Although the implementation of protection against fluctuations is immediate and results are quick, the reduction of fluctuations is usually a slow process whose effect is realized in the medium and long term. For example, the approaches for managing quality and process control according to Deming (1986) require a change in the thinking of most people in an organization. Implementing such approaches and observing significant results take considerable time, even years. Let us now examine approaches to reducing fluctuations:

- *Reducing response time.* Reducing a system's response time allows for a better prediction of demand that, in turn, allows a significant reduction of fluctuations in the system. In addition, the shorter the response time of the process, the smaller its standard deviation. For example, purchased goods arrive on an average of every eight weeks, with a standard deviation of plus or minus one week. The firm can protect against a late arrival of materials by creating a week's safety inventory through ordering a week before the original order. If response time is reduced to eight days, purchases would arrive on the average of every eight days with a standard deviation of plus or minus one day. Fluctuations will naturally be smaller, and so will the required level of safety stock.
- *Sharing information with customers and suppliers.* Sharing information reduces uncertainty. A customer providing his or her supplier with the demand forecast reduces the supplier's uncertainty and allows the supplier to obtain raw materials, plan personnel needs, and the like. Even a forecast that will materialize only 70 percent of the time but that will be periodically updated may provide important information to the supplier. Improving the performance of the supplier benefits the customer by reducing his or her fluctuations.

• *Creating a common core for several products or services (mush-room effect).* Producing or providing service for every product or service separately, as depicted in Figure 14.8, requires separate planning of resources (and raw materials) for every line. Creating a common core for several products (mushroom effect), as shown in Figure 14.9, allows the variation in the planning of resources and raw

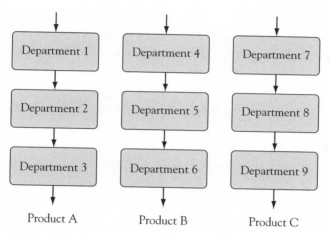

Figure 14.8. A Separate Line for Every Product.

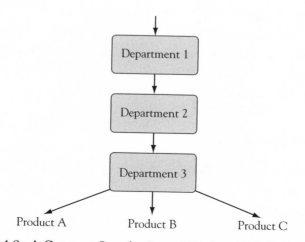

Figure 14.9. A Common Core for Several Products (Mushroom Effect).

materials to be reduced. In service organizations, this translates into a more flexible and versatile service.

• *Standardizing components and raw materials.* Standardization of raw materials and components used by the firm reduces the variability in work processes and also allows lower levels of inventory.

• *Uniting finished goods warehouses.* The variation of overall demand for finished goods stored in one central warehouse is smaller than the sum of demand variations if the finished goods were stored in several decentralized warehouses. This allows the reduction of shortages and the amount of conveyance among warehouses.

• *Using a single buffer for the entire project using the "critical chain" approach.* Using a common buffer for all project activities reduces, on average, the response time of the project along with the variance around the finishing date.

• *Reducing overspecification and overdesign.* Overspecification and overdesign cause an increase in the project time to completion and time to market. They also increase the variance in the number of development cycles and increase fluctuations in the development department.

• *Improving quality and process control.* Quality improvement and process control contribute significantly to the reduction of fluctuations. These methods are described in Chapter 17.

• *Working with small working batches and small "working packages."* Working with small working batches allows for a more continuous process with less WIP, a shorter response time, and as a result, smaller fluctuations.

Chapter Summary

Managing fluctuations is an important issue that must be considered both for planning a service or producing a product and for routine operation with the organization's resources. Fluctuations that are not properly managed may turn noncritical resources into bottlenecks, thus increasing response time, decreasing throughput, and increasing the amount of work in process. Fluctuations can be managed by protection and reduction activities.

There is no doubt that reducing fluctuations, especially through the use of quality management and process control, contributes to the output of an organization and to enhancing its value. However, its implementation is more difficult, and the results are achieved only in the medium or long term while requiring the involvement of most players in the system. It is not surprising that many quality improvement programs do not achieve their goals because of these difficulties. On the other hand, protecting against fluctuations, especially through approaches of management by constraints, is not sufficient, even though results are obtained in the short term.

Combining both approaches seems to be the right solution: starting the implementation of improvements by management by constraints, and in parallel, starting the implementation of quality management approaches. In the case of implementing steps for improvement, it is safe to say that "quality comes second."

15

The Evils of Traditional Cost Accounting

Objective

- Understand why traditional cost accounting may lead organizations to inadequate decisions

Loss of Relevance of Traditional Cost Accounting

Traditional cost accounting lost relevance back in the 1980s (Goldratt and Cox, 1986; Goldratt, 1990; Johnson and Kaplan, 1987). Traditional cost-accounting methods were developed in the 1920s in leading U.S. firms and were suitable for the production environment of those days: mass production of a limited number of products, using "economies of scale" and learning curves. Direct labor wages were a major component in costs and were considered real variable costs, taking into considerations the labor relations at that time. The indirect costs were low, and assigning them to products based on direct wages (or another volume-based variable like machine hours) was a reasonable approximation for making business decisions such as continued production of a product, investment decisions, buy-or-make decisions, and so on. For example, the pricing of one unit of product A was as follows:

Materials	$10
Direct labor	4
Overhead allocation	2
Total product cost	$16

In the business environment of the past, the traditional cost accounting allowed the breakdown of business outcomes at profit centers by individual product and preparing a balance sheet for each product separately. One could make decisions about one product (for example, increasing or decreasing production, using subcontractors) without concurrently checking the effect of the decisions on other products. This is the "separation principle," which created a convenient decision-making tool for management.

Decisions regarding a product, based on the separation principle, required knowing only the data relevant for this specific product. For example, if the market price for product A was only $13, then a decision about ceasing its production was obvious (compared with the above-listed production cost of $16). If a subcontractor would be willing to produce the product for $12, the make-or-buy decision would again be easy. In another situation, if the market price was $22 per unit, then traditional cost accounting, which is based on the "product cost," provided a good answer for decision makers.

Several factors responsible for the loss of relevancy of traditional cost accounting are described below.

Changes in the Relative Weight of the Indirect Costs

When traditional cost accounting was created in the 1920s, indirect costs were 5 to 10 percent of production costs. Today the indirect costs (overheads) constitute 20 to 80 percent of the total cost of a product. The bulk of this increase comes from costs related to operations support (planning, operations control, scheduling, engineering, quality control), information systems, the marketing force, and the managers of finance and human resources. The weight of the traditional fixed indirect costs of production (for example, depreciation, insurance, property taxes) has remained stable over time.

Changes in the Character of Salary Costs

In the past, direct labor costs were a *variable expense*. Today direct wages are mainly a *fixed cost* in the short and medium terms. However, it is still accounting-wise customary to assign the indirect costs based on direct wages, causing severe distortions.

Expanding Variety of Services and Products

Today's services and products are congruent with customers' needs and preferences. Technological development, along with the desire to adapt services and products to customers, has brought about a large increase in the variety of products, services, and treatments available today. The competitive need to expand the variety of services and products presents a managerial challenge: how to expand the variety while maintaining the advantages of the organization whose operations are focused. The cost-accounting systems must provide relevant information. Traditional cost accounting does not provide answers to the challenges of production complexity, development of prototypes, and providing a variety of services.

Not Distinguishing Between Bottlenecks and Nonbottlenecks

Today there is a clear distinction between resources that are bottlenecks and noncritical resources. The noncritical resources have built-in protective capacity that should protect the system against external fluctuations in demand, internal fluctuations resulting from malfunctions, and the like. Traditional cost accounting does not recognize this distinction.

The Dominance of Financial Accounting

The sophistication of capital markets and the stricter rules for financial reporting have led in recent decades to research and regulation in financial accounting, with emphasis on financial reporting.

Managerial accounting, however, has remained virtually at a stand-still and is considered only a secondary supportive system. When resources are channeled into managerial improvement, the financial manager (who is frequently also responsible for the information systems) will usually prefer to invest in financial accounting tools needed for reporting to a stock exchange of the Internal Revenue Service, rather than investing in managerial accounting (for example, decision-support measurement tools).

Loss of Relevance: Examples

The following examples taken from health care systems illustrate how traditional cost accounting has lost its relevance.

"It Costs Us More"

A large pharmaceutical company bought a new machine at a cost of $2 million. This machine replaced an old, labor-intensive line. It produced high-quality products in short response times and in sufficient quantities to meet all local market demand, all at a capacity utilization not exceeding 60 percent. The return on investment was less than two years. The cost of producing a unit of the product was calculated by the accountants as follows:

Raw materials	$10
Direct labor	2
Overhead	8
Total cost	$20

A foreign customer wanted to purchase 10 percent of the machine's output for $16 per unit. Even though the customer was from a totally different geographical region and even though he would have sold the product under a different name and for a different use, management refused to sell, claiming "It costs us more" and "We can't sell a product at a loss." The situation of considering costs that are not relevant for making decisions is well known and has been discussed in the literature for decades. However, many managers still use total cost data for decision making.

"Big Batches"

A new CEO immediately pushed to reduce the product cost. The average production batch size (which was congruent with the market) was ten units. Production resources were at excess capacity. Setup time was two hours, and the marginal time to produce one unit was one-quarter hour. The average time (T) to produce one unit in a batch size of ten is calculated as follows:

$$T(10) = \frac{2 + (0.25 \times 10)}{10} = \frac{2 + 2.5}{10} = \frac{4.5}{10} = 0.45 \text{ hours per unit}$$

To reduce the cost per unit (which is a local measure that has no business meaning), management decided to work with batches of one hundred units to capitalize on economies of scale:

$$T(100) = \frac{2 + (0.25 \times 100)}{100} = \frac{2 + 25}{100} = \frac{27}{100} = 0.27 \text{ hours per unit}$$

Indeed, the conclusions from such calculations were that significant savings were achieved, and the cost per unit decreased. Readers will note that production costs did not decrease at all. Because of increased work-in-process (WIP) inventory, the indirect costs increased, along with finished goods inventory, with all their ramifications.

"Efficient Production"

A public company decided to make production more efficient. It realized that the overhead multiplier is 6.2 (for every dollar spent on direct labor in production, there is an overhead of $6.20). The product cost was calculated as follows:

Raw materials	$40
Direct labor	10
Overhead	62
Total product cost	$112

The desire to make production efficient brought about a drastic reduction in direct labor and interfered with the company's bottle-neck. After a 30 percent reduction in direct labor, the cost of the product was

Raw materials	$40.00
Direct labor	7.00
Overhead	43.40
Total product cost	$90.40

The company was thrilled with its "savings" despite the reduced production throughput. Moreover, the company shared the cost reduction with the customers by offering them an additional 10 percent discount.

"Savings"

A certain department in a company had a temporary personnel shortage. The manager of the department asked a colleague, the manager of another department with excess personnel, for help. The colleague agreed to transfer some people for the needed time but demanded compensation for the full cost of the people. The manager eventually decided to hire outside help at a lower cost. The result: the company increased its expenses while the excess workers remained idle and received full pay.

Chapter Summary

Classical cost accounting lost its relevance because the underlying assumptions that are its base are no longer valid, as seen in Table 15.1.

Table 15.1. Loss of Relevance of the Assumptions Underlying Traditional Cost Accounting.

Expense	Beginning of Twentieth Century	Today
Overhead (indirect expenses) (%)	<5	20 to 80
Direct labor	Real variable cost	Fixed cost
Resources	Ability to adjust personnel	Coexistence of bottlenecks and noncritical resources (having excess capacity)

The conclusions from our analysis can be summarized as follows:

• The assumptions of traditional cost accounting, which were relevant at the beginning of the twentieth century, are usually no longer valid for analyzing costs of both industrial organizations and health care and service organizations.

• To allow better control and to assist decision making, improvements should be made in operations, marketing, sales, development, and providing service, not necessarily by focusing on accuracy of the data for costing products and services. The use of traditional cost accounting as a basis for decision making can lead to wrong managerial decisions.

For proper decision making, other tools are required. In the next chapter, we present alternatives to traditional cost accounting that are appropriate for the modern business environment.

16

Marketing, Costing, and Pricing Considerations in Decision-Making Processes

Objective

- Understand how the global decision-making (GDM) method can be used as an effective tool for making decisions

Managerial Decision Making

To deal with the irrelevancy of traditional cost accounting and to aid managerial decision making, two approaches have been developed in recent years: activity-based costing and throughput accounting.

Activity-Based Costing

The activity-based cost-accounting method is actually a refinement and improvement of classical cost accounting ("absorbing accounting") and was first introduced by Cooper and Kaplan (1988). Activity-based cost accounting analyzes the indirect costs and assigns them in sophisticated and precise methods across the various services or products.

Throughput Accounting

Throughput accounting is an updated version of contribution accounting that was introduced in the 1940s. Throughput accounting was offered by Goldratt (1990) as a managerial decision-making tool. In this chapter, we discuss the basics of throughput accounting and improve on it by adding a structured method (global decision making, or GDM) and simple tools that will aid in managerial decision making.

We feel that activity-based costing only partially aids decision-making processes and is in fact using cost allocation that is somewhat arbitrary and not relevant (Eden and Ronen, 2002). The resources of an organization are a critical factor in decision-making processes regarding pricing, investment, make or buy, and the like. We have to distinguish between two situations:

- Decision making in a resource-constrained environment (resource constraint)

- Decision making in an excess capacity environment (market constraint)

Decision Making in a Resource-Constrained Environment

Today's competitive business environment is usually an environment with excess capacity in operational resources or services, and the market is a buyers' market. However, there are many situations where an organization is constrained by a bottleneck. These bottlenecks include departments that are permanent bottlenecks (like development or marketing and sales) and when a bottleneck results from a shortage of an expensive resource, a shortage of skilled professionals, peak or seasonal periods, and events of temporary or continual shortage of raw materials or critical resources.

In a resource-constrained environment, managers face the following decision problems:

- *Problems of product mix:* A resource-constrained environment cannot produce *all* products with market potential or deliver all possible services to the customer. System performance is limited by its constraints, and a resource constraint forces managers to decide on a product or service mix: on the one hand, which products to manufacture and which services to sell and, on the other hand, which products or services to exclude or discontinue.

• *Make-or-buy decisions:* A make-or-buy decision is a common managerial decision problem. Decisions to use subcontractors require strategic and tactical judgment. The advantage of subcontractors is the lifting of the resource constraint, which allows the expansion of the effective manufacturing or service ability of the organization. The important decision is which jobs to perform in-house (make) and which to purchase from subcontractors (buy) while considering system resources.

• *Pricing decisions:* At which price should a product or service be offered to the market? How should a product that passes through the bottleneck be priced, and at what price should a product or service that does not pass through it be sold (free goods)?

• *Decisions on stopping production or ceasing service:* Decisions on stopping production or ceasing a service must be made from the perspective of the well-being of the whole organization (globally) while considering system constraints. As we have seen, decisions based on traditional cost accounting can lead to system failure.

• *Decisions to introduce a new product or service line:* These decisions must be made from a global perspective, making wise use of information regarding system resources and understanding the effect on the critical resources.

• *Investment decisions:* The best investment decisions are those that enhance the value of the firm. GDM supports the increase of throughput, the reduction of operating expenses, or the increase in the difference between them. In the case of a system constraint, controlled investments that relieve the bottleneck are usually the ones that will lead to increased profits and value enhancement for the firm.

• *Decision on acceptance and pricing of projects:* A project environment, which is common to high-tech industries, is usually an environment with constraints on development resources. The manager must decide which projects to prefer and how to price them.

• *Decisions on bidding for contracts:* As we have seen before, managers who use traditional cost accounting cannot distinguish between work hours of excess capacity resources and work hours of constrained resources. The strategic and tactical tools that are presented in this chapter will help make decisions on bidding for contracts.

• *Decisions or product differentiation and market segmentation:* Product differentiation and market segmentation are important marketing tools. In many industries (for example, cosmetics, automotive), segmentation and differentiation have been customary for years. However, many organizations have yet to capitalize on the differentiation and segmentation potential. Smart use of the critical resource can lead to better segmentation and differentiation decisions.

The Tools

Several tools help decision-making processes. The following are suitable both for a resource-constrained environment and one with excess capacity (market constraint):

1. Global performance measures
2. The GDM method (see below)
3. The measurements profile
4. A cost-utilization (CUT) diagram (discussed in Chapter 4 and below)

An additional tool is unique for a resource-constrained environment:

5. Specific contribution

The GDM Method for Decision Making: Adding Strategic Considerations

The GDM method (Geri and Ronen, 2005) is simple and practical. It helps in making decisions on pricing, make or buy, stopping production of a product, or shutting down a line of products or services, among others. The three steps of the method are as follows:

1. Make a global economic decision from the perspective of the CEO.
2. Make strategic considerations.
3. Change, if needed, local performance measures.

Step 1: GDM from the CEO's Perspective

The decision should be such that it would achieve the maximal contribution to the organization's objective function and should reflect the CEO's perspective. The decision will use two tools we have introduced: measurements profile and a CUT diagram.

Step 2: Strategic Considerations

Strategic considerations relate to the long run and to considerations that involve intangible benefits. Step 1 generates an economic decision. Now the manager can make strategic considerations that may change the global economic decision, and he or she can calculate what the strategic issues would cost the organization. Decisions are frequently made without in-depth analysis, with the claim that it was a strategic decision. The strategic considerations of management are important, but they will be more appropriate if they carry a price tag.

Step 3: Changes to Local Performance Measures

Local performance measures frequently distort the decision-making process. A manager occasionally prefers to make a wrong decision but one that would maximize his or her local or personal performance measure, rather than a decision that would better serve the organization. Hence, there is a managerial necessity to examine and adapt the local performance measures to maximize the organizational objective function. The use of local measures such as profit per product or service, cost per service or product, or number of units produced or served may distort decisions, and therefore, these measures should be changed.

Decision Making in an Excess Capacity Environment

The GDM method is valid both in a resource-constrained environment (a resource constraint) and in an excess capacity environment (market constraint).

The following example highlights the use of the GDM method in make-or-buy decisions in situations of excess capacity:

Dilemma: A large health maintenance organization (HMO) operates a testing laboratory as an independent profit center. The lab has excess testing capacity. However, because of the highly skilled and specialized lab technicians and staff, the HMO is inclined to keep a critical mass of the existing lab staff and not to sell any of its equipment. The HMO needs to perform one million tests in the coming year, which would still leave the lab at excess capacity. The lab charges $3 per blood test. The HMO has the possibility of "buying" blood tests from a local hospital for $2 per test. The variable costs per test are 50 cents. The HMO decided to buy the tests from the hospital because of the lower total testing costs and for long-term strategic considerations that relate to the relationship with this and other hospitals.

Analysis: In a world of local performance measures, it seems reasonable for the HMO to turn the work over to an external hospital laboratory (a buy decision) rather than perform it in house (make) because this would be $1 million better for the balance sheet. Seemingly, the HMO saves $1 million by making this decision. Actually, the HMO spent $2.5 million out of pocket, and the fixed costs of the lab that it owns were not affected. (The variable costs would have been incurred in both cases.)

Let us now examine the decision in the case example by the GDM method:

- *Make a global economic decision from the CEO's perspective.* The CUT diagram for the testing laboratory is presented in Figure 16.1. This is a situation with excess capacity, and if the HMO-owned lab will perform the tests, the picture will be similar.

Table 16.1 presents the measurements profile for the decision. The throughput of an organization is defined as the actual sales minus the real variable costs of these sales. Thus, the costs paid to the subcontractor in a buy decision will reduce the firm's throughput by $2.5 million. The operational expenses (in conditions of excess capacity in the HMO lab) will not change. The total cost for salaries, rent, and machine maintenance will remain the same, whether the work will be done in-house or outside of the company.

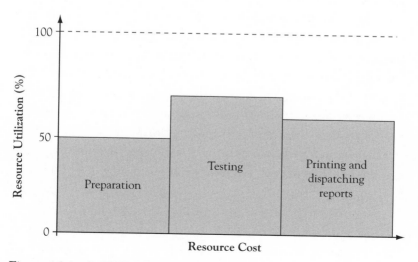

Figure 16.1. A CUT Diagram for Blood Tests.

Table 16.1. Measurements Profile for a Make-or-Buy Decision.

Measurement	Make	Buy
Throughput (T)	X	X –$2.5 million
Operating expenses (OE)	Y	Y
Inventory (I)	–	–
Response time (RT)	–	–
Quality (Q)	–	–
Due date performance (DDP)	–	–

Key: X is the HMO's total monetary throughput if the work is done within the HMO. Y is its operating expenses.

The bottom line is that giving the work to the subcontractor will reduce profits.

With respect to the other measures, every measure must be dealt with separately, considering its pros and cons for each alternative. It is clear from the measurements profile that if the last four measures (inventory, response time, quality, and due date performance) are similar for the two alternatives, then the make (in-house testing) decision should be preferred to the buy (subcontracting) one.

• *Make strategic considerations.* We must take into account long-term considerations and ones that relate to intangible benefits. On the one hand, the firm may have an interest in preserving the external subcontractor in a working relation because of planned future growth of the company. On the other hand, one must consider the negative strategic implications in using a subcontractor. A subcontractor may receive important information that may help him or her become a strategic competitor. At this stage, we know the financial implications of each alternative and thus may make the decision on economic grounds.

In many situations, the strategic consideration may include the following question: Is the relevant technology a *core competence* of the organization? Figure 16.2 presents the "core competence matrix" that assists in making a make-or-buy decision. It combines the

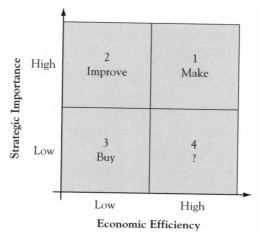

Figure 16.2. A Core Competence Matrix.

strategic dimension of the technology and the efficiency dimension of the relevant department. A department situated in quadrants 1 or 2 in the matrix has strategic importance to the organization: this is its core competence. The jobs of these departments should be performed in-house—for example, a department for developments in a high-tech firm, or project management in a company that does overseas construction.

The tasks of departments in quadrant 1 should be performed in-house. Departments in quadrant 2 have core competence that should be kept within the organization, but they should not operate at low efficiency. One must find ways to improve the performance of such departments, make them more efficient, and shift them to quadrant 1. Jobs of departments in quadrant 3 should be sent outside the organization to a subcontractor or to outsourcing services—for example, dining or cleaning services in a hospital. They do not have core competence and are not efficient. Decisions regarding departments in quadrant 4 will be evaluated individually according to the current strategy of the organization.

Assigning jobs to subcontractors is a strategic decision of management. An attempt to resolve the make-or-buy decision on local economic considerations may be detrimental to the organization. A decision based on the economic wisdom of letting market forces dictate actions empowers internal customers within the organization to make the make-or-buy decisions. This approach allows management to disengage itself from the problem, perhaps leading to a "drying out" of strategic technological departments. Such an approach will also prevent future investments needed to preserve the technological ability of strategically important departments with cutting-edge technology and information.

A policy of performing jobs outside the organization only because of local economic considerations may bring about the loss of core competence and a loss of clear strategic advantages.

A hospital used subcontractors for all its information technology needs, including billing and patient records. Over the years, the entire body of knowledge that related to these systems was completely outside the hospital. This created a strategic and economic dependence on the subcontractors and limited the influence the hospital had on future development of information technology products.

A firm specializing in the production of testing equipment realized that the production of its products became rather standard. They outsourced production to a multinational firm in Asia, allowing considerable savings in production costs. The realized savings encouraged management to outsource sales and marketing as well. Giving away strategic marketing abilities to foreign hands resulted in a steep drop in sales and ultimately bankruptcy.

Management and control are strategic capabilities in many organizations. Giving those abilities away makes an organization vulnerable to loss of control of its operations.

- *Change, if needed, local performance measures.* Factors that delay reaching the right decision in this situation are local performance measures such as the hourly rate and project profits. One must aspire to change them. The measurement of project profit can be refined by using an external alternative transfer price. Another possibility is to make the production unit into a cost center (instead of a profit center), which management will want to keep in-house for strategic reasons (Horngren, Foster, and Datar, 2000).

Decisions on Stopping Production or Ceasing Service

We will now illustrate the use of the GDM method for a problem of deciding to stop production of a product. The same technique can be used to analyze the cessation of some service. Suppose management is wondering whether to stop production of a certain diagnostic kit. The production line used for this product is at excess capacity, and in the coming year there is no planned effective use of this capacity. The market price of the kit is $4.00, and the production costs (by traditional cost accounting) are as follows:

Raw materials	$2.00
Packaging	0.50
Direct labor	0.75
Processing	0.31
Depreciation	0.20
Indirect costs	1.10
Total product cost	$4.86

Projected sales of the kit are ten thousand units per month. According to traditional cost accounting, the company is losing 86 cents for every unit sold. As a result, management is considering stopping production of this kit. It should be noted that the company will not lay off workers if they close the line because they are needed for other tasks. Let us examine the situation using the GDM method.

• *Make a global economic decision from the CEO's perspective:* The CEO should draw a CUT diagram for the production line and consider the various alternatives. The CUT diagram reveals excess capacity.

Let us examine in Table 16.2 the measurements profile of the two alternatives. Throughput will be reduced by $15,000 because the selling price is $4.00 per unit, and the variable costs are $2.50:

$$10,000 \ (\$4.00 - \$2.50) = \$15,000$$

The real variable costs in the production are the raw materials and packaging. Some of the processing costs can also be considered variable (energy and parts). The manager will consider the other variables as needed.

The fixed costs are not about to change. Hence, the economic decision should be to continue manufacturing. The contribution of sales in this case helps cover the fixed costs and should not be given up.

• *Make strategic considerations:* By stopping production of the kit, the important strategic considerations are, Will the stoppage of

Table 16.2. Measurements Profile for the Production Example.

Measurement	Continue Production	Stop Production
Throughput (T)	X	X –$15,000
Operating expenses (OE)	Y	Y
Inventory (I)	—	—
Response time (RT)	—	—
Quality (Q)	—	—
Due date performance (DDP)	—	—

Key: X is the organization's total monetary throughput. Y is its operating expenses in case production is continued.

sales negatively affect the firm's reputation? Will competitors capture the market share given up by the firm? In any case, step 1 of the method will present to management the cost of each strategic decision.

• *Change, if needed, local performance measures:* If a department manager's performance is measured by a local balance sheet of a product line, this measure must be changed. Performance measures that take throughput into account could be an appropriate substitute.

What to Do with Excess Capacity in Production and Service Resources

In the modern service and production environment, excess of operational capacity is widely spread. The question is, what should be done with this excess? Let us consider the following service mix example: A private medical center is considering what price to charge for a new homeopathic service. The variable costs (mainly drugs) are $55 per visit. The other costs are fixed, and the medical center has excess capacity that allows serving one million customers annually. The marketing consultants envision three scenarios for market demand (Table 16.3), and the demand curve is represented graphically in Figure 16.3. The natural solution is to choose the price that will maximize contribution. However, the maximal contribution will be if the service will be offered at each of the three prices: segment the market to those charged $100, those charged $80, and patients who will be charged $60.

Let us examine this example using the GDM method:

Table 16.3. Demand as a Function of Price.

Scenario	Price per Visit ($)	Demand (patients per year)
A	100	100,000
B	80	200,000
C	60	500,000

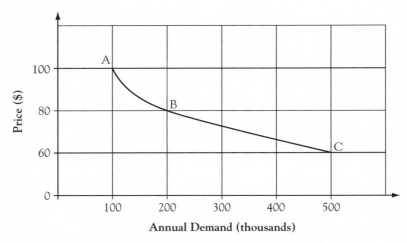

Figure 16.3. Demand Curve for the Service Mix Example.

• *Make a global economic decision from the CEO's perspective:* We will first examine the problem using the measurements profile shown in Table 16.4. The global economic decision is to sell the service at three differential prices. This will yield the highest contribution to the medical center, hence the highest profit.

• *Make strategic considerations:* Long-term strategic considerations place several threats on the organization when selling at all three prices.

When prices in the market are falling, selling the service to C customers can lead to a price drop for A and B customers.

The salespeople, feeling that the margin of sales is only the variable costs, will sell the service in the future to all customers at lower prices (close to $55). Salespeople always want to sell (occasionally at any price) and will justify this by the positive marginal benefit to the firm.

An A customer will find out that the service is sold to market segment C at a lower price and will demand the lower price as well. In addition, the A customer will feel cheated.

Table 16.4. Measurements Profile for the Service Mix Example.

Measurement	No Service	Sell A	Sell B	Sell C	Sell at All Prices
Throughput (T) ($ millions)	X	X + 4.5	X + 5.0	X + 2.5	X + 8.5
Operating expenses (OE)	Y	Y	Y	Y	Y
Inventory (I)	—	—	—	—	—
Response time (RT)	—	—	—	—	—
Quality (Q)	—	—	—	—	—
Due date performance (DDP)	—	—	—	—	—

Key: X is the medical center's throughput while no homeopathic service is offered. Y is the operating expenses in that case.

A and B customers may demand to get the lower rates even for their past visits. They may now demand lower prices for other clinic services.

There is the danger that the excess capacity will quickly be filled up with services sold at cheap prices. These dangers can be overcome by *product differentiation and market segmentation*. The services will be sold in different forms to different market segments, priced at the perceived value of these segments. Many industries have specialized in market segmentation and product differentiation, and other industries have not done so. An airline passenger flying first class may pay up to five times more than a passenger in economy class, and both of them feel they are getting their money's worth. Moreover, two passengers sitting next to each other in economy class may have paid different prices for the same flight because their tickets may be of a different class, reflecting restrictions, and so forth. The electronics industry differentiates products by performance or by brand names that reflect the perceived value of the products to the customers.

The high-tech industry differentiates products by performance mainly by downgrading performance. The automotive industry differentiates by model type (two-door, four-door, coupe, sedan, station wagon), the number of features, type of transmission, and manufacturer (General Motors has several brand names, such as Buick, Chevrolet, and Cadillac).

In most cases, the cost differential in providing differential services or producing different products is small relative to the price differences customers are willing to pay. Therefore, the dimension of differentiation will include the following:

- Performance

- Brand name

- Size

- Quality

- Reliability

- Quantity

- Repetitiveness of service or product (for example, one or frequent clinic visits)

- Seasonality (in season or out of season)

- Packaging

- Warranty

- Service level

- Geographical differentiation

- Response times

Correct product or service differentiation and market segmentation can provide answers to the potential dangers of upper-market segments pushing prices down.

- *Change, if needed, local performance measures:* Local performance measures such as price per unit may lead to failure that will prevent correct product differentiation and market segmentation.

Chapter Summary

The GDM method presented in this chapter is a simple and efficient tool for making decisions. It bypasses the need to determine product cost or product profit, whose use could be problematic. This method is good for pricing decisions, make-or-buy decisions, pricing a new product or service, stopping production or a service, determining transfer prices or bid prices, determining product mix, and evaluating investments.

With all the benefits provided by this method, we must not ignore its danger, which is the lack of threshold. Traditional cost accounting, with all of its "lack of common sense," determines a cost threshold. The disadvantages of a threshold are known: it is arbitrary and leads to loss of business opportunities. However, it provides a barrier to the pressure from salespeople to sell more and more at any cost while causing attrition in prices.

Users of the method must maintain a constant mechanism for determining a "performance threshold" by management for every product or family of products or services. This threshold will be determined by market prices, availability of resources, and strategic considerations. Such a mechanism requires a high level of management that enables differential treatment of products or services.

An organization that uses this method must have a common language among people in finance, marketing, development, and operations. Understanding the managerial approaches behind this method will result in better decisions at both strategic and tactical levels.

17

Quality Management and Process Control

Objectives

- Understand the need to measure and improve quality

- Learn how to break common quality myths

One of the major breakthroughs in management over the past decades was in the area of quality management and process control. Quality is today one of the most important factors in the competitive environment of any organization.

Poor quality has an adverse effect on the value of an organization by contributing both to a decrease in income and an increase in expenses. On the other hand, good quality has positive effects on income and expenses.

We view quality as an important value driver and as a tool for improving processes, products, and services. In this chapter, we present quality and process control in a goal-oriented business approach. We show that good quality and a reduction of expenses can be achieved simultaneously.

What Is Quality?

There are many definitions of *quality*, and we will relate the more prominent ones, that is, the operational approach, the economic approach, the centrality of the customer, and the uniformity or consistency approach.

Operational Approach

The *operational approach,* characterized by Crosby (1979), states that quality means *conformance to requirements.* A product, service, or prototype has quality only if it conforms to the requirements dictated by the customer, the manufacturer, management, or standard of some specifications. According to this definition, there is no quality difference between a brand new Rolls Royce that meets customer requirements or a Volkswagen Beetle (the older model) that was manufactured to meet all its required specifications. Service provided at a fast-food chain like McDonald's can be considered of high quality if it meets standards of waiting times, service rules, and food preparation procedures as specified by the company. The first step in creating quality according to Crosby is to *define requirements.* We often come to realize that services or products do not have well-defined requirements. New products are occasionally developed with incomplete specifications, resulting in many development cycles and delays in project completion.

Economic Approach

The *economic approach* to quality is defined by Schonberger (1986) in two dimensions that reflect quality of an organization and are closely related:

- Achieving a minimal "garbage plant"
- Doing it right the first time

The *garbage plant:* all activities that do not add value to the customer, the product, the service, or the process.

The economic approach considers the labor hours, money, and materials that are wasted on repairs, rework, errors, customer compensation for a bad service or product, and time devoted to solving these problems. This is also the noneffective time of specialists and marketing and sales personnel. The garbage plant refers to the "nonconformance quality costs" that take away dozens of percentages of workers' or managers' time.

Following are examples of garbage plants:

In the billing department of a health maintenance organization (HMO), it turned out that many of the billing people spend a lot of time correcting billing errors.

In the operating room (OR) of a hospital, much time of surgeons and nurses as well as OR time was wasted because of patients arriving with incomplete kits, thus delaying or canceling operations.

In a large hospital lab, several technicians spent most of their time looking for and correcting problems.

The marketing personnel for a large HMO report that 40 to 60 percent of their time is ineffective because of repeated or cancelled meetings and incomplete kits.

The customer service department of a large insurance company reports that dozens of workers spend hours on the phone trying to resolve problems that arose from mistakes or ambiguities in insurance policies.

In a certain restaurant, about 10 percent of customers received the wrong dish simply because orders were not written down and the waiter tried to memorize them. This resulted in delays in food delivery, food that had to be discarded, wasted time of waiters and cooks, and unhappy customers, some of whom would not return to the restaurant.

Much of the garbage plant can be avoided. It is clear that we cannot always provide a service or produce a product with zero defects. However, by reducing the garbage plant from 50 to 30 percent, for example, one can achieve economic advantages and enhance an organization's value.

Performing a task *right the first time* means that *every* step in the process of performing a task is successfully completed the first time around without failures or quality problems.

When a task is done right the first time, there is no need to redo any of the steps.

Centrality of the Customer

The *centrality of the customer* approach is derived from Juran's definition of quality (1989). Juran, one of the founding fathers of quality theory, claims that one of the most important dimensions of quality is "fitness to use." This fitness emphasizes the centrality of the customer. The customer is the one who sets the standards; thus, the whole organization, including products, services, prototypes, and workers, should be subordinated to customers' requirements. The product or service must be fit for customers' use. Juran views the work processes as a chain of *internal suppliers that work to fulfill the needs and requirements of the internal customers*. Alongside this, every element in the value chain of the organization should view itself as serving the *external customer*.

Uniformity Approach

Taguchi (1986), an engineer and one of the founders of modern quality theory, emphasized *consistency and minimal variance* as critical components of quality. According to this approach, a service or product that is offered with minimum variation and uniform and consistent performance is testimony to a *controlled process*.

In service organizations, uniformity or consistency means a process that repeats itself again and again with minimal variation over time.

In the health care system, waiting times in a clinic are considered one measure of service quality. If patients wait once for ten minutes and sometimes two hours, the resulting variation is problematic. If they have alternatives, such inconsistency in the level of service may drive patients to the competition.

In the McDonald's fast-food chain, consistency is one of the key dimensions of quality. This means a consistently high level of service that conforms to requirements of time standards, performance, and service. In every McDonald's in the world, a customer knows what to expect and will get the same quality burgers and fries that are produced using the *same* methods. This consistency is a value enhancer for the chain that produces a reputation that brings customers back again and again.

An example where lack of consistency had severely negative effects is the Howard Johnson's restaurant chain. For years, customers knew what to expect at any restaurant in the chain. At some point, variation among restaurants developed, and the lack of consistency in what customers were receiving eventually led to the disappearance of this restaurant chain.

In production, consistency means having good control over a process, meaning the capability of producing the same product again and again, even thousands of times, regardless of other factors that may introduce variability into the system. Such factors include

- Suppliers of raw materials

- Raw materials and components

- Workers

- Production specifications

- Equipment and computerization

The fact that an organization is able to maintain consistency and minimal variability despite the above factors that introduce "noise" and changes is testimony to the fact that it is able to achieve near-complete process control. This control assures the continual production of the same product at the same quality over time.

We presented here four of the more popular definitions of quality. There are other definitions of quality that describe quality as meeting customer expectations or even exceeding them. Other definitions break quality down into several dimensions like reliability, performance, perceived quality, response time, and life cycle.

As we shall see later in this chapter, improving processes of service, production, and development yields improvement along any definition of quality. An organization that realizes that a certain quality definition will enhance its value will take quality-improving actions to implement this specific definition.

Stages in Managing Quality and Process Control

There are three main stages in quality management and process control: no quality management, inspection, and then process control.

Stage One: The Organization Has No Quality Management and Feedback

Organizations in this stage are usually monopolistic: they lack customer awareness and feedback systems for process control and improvement. At this stage, the organization is "doing its best" and solves problems in an ad hoc manner. Customer complaints are usually answered by "we worked by the guidelines" or the customer "does not understand, is not right, and is responsible." More serious complaints are solved by apologies or gifts.

Stage Two: Inspection: Quality Control at the End of the Process

At this stage, the organization adds a function of quality control at the end of the process (inspection), performed by the quality control department, which is an independent body. These inspectors examine the final products and screen out the defective ones, as seen in Figure 17.1. There is no doubt that being in stage two with inspection (quality control) at the end of the line is preferable to being in stage one because there is some control over the outcome of the process. However, experience shows that inspection, as good as it may be, does not prevent defects. Moreover, the mere existence of a quality control department relieves responsibility from the operations people, who see the quality control people as responsible for quality. There is also the undesirable tension between personnel in the two areas. Because no preventive measures are introduced, the garbage plant continues to produce defective services and products. This approach is "open-circle control" that indeed identifies current problems but usually does not prevent future ones.

Stage Three: Process Control

Every organization wishing to survive in today's competitive environment must reach the stage of process control, the sooner the better. This stage is also referred to as *Deming's theory* (Deming, 1986). At this stage, we have "closed-loop control," which is control with feedback at constant and short intervals, as seen in Figure 17.2.

The following are the principles of process control:

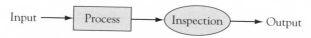

Figure 17.1. Adding Inspection at the End of the Line.

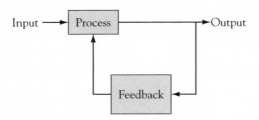

Figure 17.2. A Closed-Loop Control System.

• *The goal is continuous improvement of organizational performance:* This improvement will usually manifest itself in increasing the throughput of the organization.

• *Continuous improvement:* This reflects continuous improvement of processes. Many managerial cultures focus on the short term and on achieving immediate and one-time results. Improvement and advantages achieved by an organization will usually also be achieved by competitors in the near future. To establish a continuous competitive edge, there must be continuous improvement of processes in marketing and sales, production processes, engineering processes, and the like.

• *Emphasis on process improvement:* Quality is achieved through correct processes.

The *85-15 rule* states that 85 percent of failures are caused by inappropriate processes and are the responsibility of management. Only 15 percent of failures are the responsibility of workers.

Processes that are under management's responsibility include, among others, selection, recruitment, and training of employees; setting and measuring work processes; measuring and rewarding employees; working with complete kits; and processes of sales, marketing, pricing, and costing.

When a problem occurs in an organization, everybody is mobilized to solve it. However, in an organization that did not undergo the conceptual change in the spirit of Deming's theory, right after the problem has been solved, the unavoidable hunt for those responsible begins.

The process control approach suggests that after a problem is solved, the following question must be addressed: What was wrong in the *process* that caused the failure, and what can be changed in the process so this failure will not recur in the future?

> One of the authors of this book was seen in the emergency department (ED) of a large governmental hospital where he arrived with severe abdominal pains. After spending a while in observation, he was discharged home despite a high white blood cell count. He was not examined by a surgeon. Two days later, he was rushed to another hospital where a computed tomographic scan revealed a ruptured appendix; he was rushed to emergency surgery and luckily survived to cowrite this book! The failure was not the human error of missing the high white blood cell count but a process failure under the responsibility of management. It is not the fault of an incompetent physician but that of management that assigned only an intern and a resident for that shift.

> In a certain regional airline, planes hitting birds was a major cause of plane crashes. When the process was investigated, it turned out that bird migration repeats itself with high precision every year. As a result, corrective measures were taken to significantly reduce the number of crashes resulting from birds.

- *Preventing rather than fixing:* The major focus should be on appropriate design of the process and on measures to avoid failures.

> A large HMO is interested in investing more in prevention than in treatment of preventable conditions. As a result of this strategic decision,

the HMO initiates a campaign promoting healthier lifestyles and physical activity. They initiate free screening clinics for various conditions, and they finance sessions of aerobic exercises and other sports activities.

• *Use of data:* Process control is possible only if the organization routinely collects data on what is happening with the process and analyzes them. ("In God we trust. All others should bring data.")

• *Use of graphical tools:* The recommended control tools are process control charts, Pareto analysis, and various graphical tools (Deming, 1986). These tools enable focused and effective analysis of the data and the identification of negative phenomena that require intervention and corrective measures. The continuous improvement in work processes achieved in this way brings about value enhancement in the long run.

• *Quality management and process control by workers:* The modern approach to quality management and process control states that a person doing a job is also responsible for its quality. This requires setting initial conditions and an appropriate work environment:

• What is considered a "good" product or service must be clearly defined.

• Workers and managers must be given the tools needed to evaluate the quality of a service or product.

• Rules and procedures must be specified that will clearly define what has to be done when a failure or a defective product or service is detected.

• *The "ten-times rule":* The later the stage that a problem is detected, fixing it will be ten times more expensive.

If certain medical conditions are diagnosed early at a community clinic, the consequences can be minor. If the condition is detected only after the patient is brought to the ED, the consequences, both clinical and financial, could be magnified ten times. If the problem is detected only while the patient is hospitalized or during surgery, another tenfold harm can be expected. If the patient is discharged and the problem reappears later, the consequences could be grave (literally speaking).

Similarly, if a defective component in a medical device was detected while the incoming shipment was being inspected, fixing it would be one-tenth the cost of fixing the problem if detected during production and one one-hundredth of the cost needed to fix the problem if detected during final quality control inspection.

The ten-times rule is presented graphically in Figure 17.3. The conclusion is that most emphasis of control and inspection must be shifted toward the *beginning* of the process, rather than at the end (as is customary in stage two of quality control).

- *Participation of managers and employees:* A quality product, service, or development is achieved by a quality process when the employees and managers are part of the process and are actively

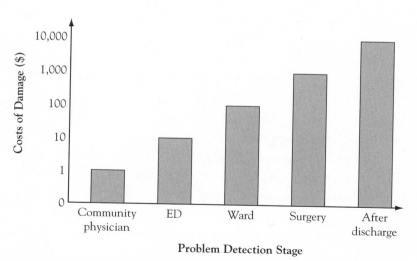

Figure 17.3. The Ten-Times Rule.

involved in the process design and control. Workers should be encouraged to be involved and should be delegated more responsibility for the quality of the work so they will feel part of the process and more committed to it. Evaluating, recognizing, and rewarding workers for their accomplishments result in quality improvement.

- *Teamwork:* A process is improved when teamwork is used to identify problems, solve them, and prevent their recurrence. Experience shows that many problems are interdepartmental problems (suppliers and internal customers), and multidisciplinary teams are effective in solving them.

- *Commitment of management:* Management must be committed to quality improvement and process control and must be involved. Quality improvement is not a stand-alone project but rather part of the tasks of an organization that manifest themselves in the budget, the work plan, and the routine control through the use of the regular tools of the organization.

- *Centrality of the customer:* The customer must be the focus of attention of all levels of an organization. In an era of excess capacity in services and production and of fierce competition, all decision making should be subordinate to the market.

- *Working with a small number of quality suppliers:* When looking globally at the long-term life-cycle cost of products and services, we realize that quality processes save money. One must work in cooperation with suppliers in a way that is based on problem identification and the goodwill of both sides to solve them. This kind of cooperation can be achieved only by working closely with a small number of quality suppliers.

It should be noted that the approach of developing mutual long-term relations with a small number of suppliers is in contrast to the approach and the statutory responsibility of most public organizations to publish offerings for bids before any substantial agreement is signed. The bidding approach can reduce costs in the short term, but it makes it difficult for an organization to maintain and assure a quality service or production process. The savings in costs are frequently offset by losses resulting from poor quality. On the other hand, we do not recommend going to the other extreme and putting all the eggs in one basket by working with a single contractor. This exposes the organization to commercial and economic risks.

Implementing Quality Improvement Processes

Quality improvement processes in organizations should be implemented using a business approach in combination with additional managerial approaches. The purpose of quality improvement in not-for-profit organizations is to improve organizational performance, and in business organizations, it is to enhance their value.

Implementing only a partial or limited quality improvement confined to areas of operations (service and production) will yield limited improvement in performance. Customers, indeed, want a high-quality product or service, but they also want fast response, reliable supply times, good performance, and services and products that are congruent with their needs, all this with competitive prices. In other words, management must evaluate the organization in a global manner as one complex entity whose components must function better. Moreover, in most organizations, profit increases that occur by improving marketing, development, and engineering are more significant than profit increases that occur by improving production processes. Unfortunately, many managers equate quality improvement with improvements in production processes or improvements in service.

Management must focus on the important issues of an organization. Critical issues must be identified by adopting a global perspective. Critical issues should be managed using effective and efficient management tools. In other words, a successful implementation of quality improvement implies combining quality improvement using Deming's approach with approaches such as management by constraints, just-in-time (JIT) approach, managerial measurement and control, the complete-kit concept, and advanced strategic approaches.

Experience shows that employing just one managerial approach yields only partial success. Quality improvement should be implemented using the following steps:

- At first, improve operational systems by implementing JIT approaches, management by constraints, measurement and control, and the complete-kit concept. This step quickly results in increased throughput, reduced response times, and quality enhancement (mainly through the reduction of work in process).
- Use quality improvement and process control methods, working with departmental and interdepartmental teams, and implement process control charts.
- Extract strategic advantages following quality improvement: turn to markets that pay more for better quality, increase prices in certain markets, and compete with lower prices in other markets. This is possible through the implementation of quality work processes, reduction of variable costs (especially raw materials), and increased throughput.

The "Throughput World" and the "Cost World"

The objective of quality improvement is to increase organizational profits, mainly through increasing throughput, by increasing contributions from increased sales and better use of raw materials. Deming (1986) believes that the objective is to increase profits and to create more jobs by increasing market share, reducing response times, adapting the product or service to the customer, and high quality. This philosophy, which focuses on increasing the throughputs of the organization, is referred to as the *throughput world* (Goldratt, 1990).

In contrast to the throughput world, there is a different philosophy whose focus is on cost reduction in the organization. This quickly translates into a desire of management to reduce the size of the workforce. This is known as the *cost world*, and it occasionally conflicts with the objectives of quality improvement. In organizations that do not have job security for workers, it will be difficult for management to involve the workforce while making changes. In many cases, the big money is made not by reducing costs but rather by increasing throughput or improving quality.

Quality Improvement Myths

Quality management and process control, according to Deming (stage three), break several myths that relate to quality management:

Myth: Quality Work Takes More Time

Reality: Quality work requires a good and structured process, and then it takes *less time*. For example, working with a complete kit in a development, sales, or production process requires fewer cycles in the process and naturally a smaller time investment and shorter cycle time.

Myth: Quality Costs More Money

Reality: High-quality work and a quality process cost *less money* because they result in less rework and fewer cycles, and they *reduce* the garbage plant. Thus, quality costs less and contributes to higher profit. Many customers are willing to pay a premium for quality services or products.

Myth: It Is Not Possible to Provide a Quality Service or Quality Product in Large Quantities

Reality: It is possible to provide quality service and produce a quality product even in large quantities if the process is *good, consistent, and reliable*. For example, customers of a cell phone company may receive quality service if the company develops a quality process: a good software system that supports the call center and provides answers to most queries and a quality process of selecting, training, and controlling the employees.

Chapter Summary

Quality improvement and process control are means that an organization must employ to survive and thrive in a competitive environment. Organizations that will not meet the required quality standard, which rises year after year, will not survive. Organizations that will use quality improvement as a competitive tool can enhance their value.

Quality improvement, in combination with approaches detailed in Part Two of this book—management by constraints, the JIT approach, the complete kit, and the Pareto rule—can all enhance organizational value without substantial (if at all) financial investments and enable the organization to do more with existing resources.

Part III

Strategy and Value Creation

18

Creating Value for Health Care Organizations

Objective

- Understand the value-focused management approach to increasing the value of a health care organization by increasing its cash flow or, in a not-for-profit organization, to improving its performance

One of the major problems faced by managers is how to initiate the process of enhancing value or improving performance and what priorities to set on the various possible improvements. For example, should they first perform improvements in the emergency department (ED), the operating rooms (ORs), or perhaps in the laboratories or imaging services? Should management focus on improvements in the internal medicine wards, or should they focus on logistics or purchasing?

A manager in a health care organization cannot afford to spend more than 10 percent of his or her time on pursuing improvements. This is the nature of the role, which makes managers spend most of their time on managing current and emergency situations, occasionally involving risking human life. The complexity of management and technology inevitably forces managers to spend most of their time on current issues.

There is no doubt that the manager of every ward or department (ED, surgery) can and should make significant improvements in that ward or department. However, the major problems of organizations are interdepartmental ones, and only proactive efforts by management can lead to improvements. For example, improvements in the ED cannot be implemented by the chief of that department alone because the work process also involves imaging and laboratory services, consultants, and the inpatient wards.

Value Creation from Managerial Activities

In this chapter, we present a holistic and global approach to where management should focus based on the importance of the improvement and ease of implementing it. The goal of an organization is to increase its value for shareholders. The goal of the management, therefore, is to bring about a constant creation of value for the shareholders, and it is therefore incumbent on management to constantly strive to achieve this goal. Increasing shareholders' value usually results in better job security, financial benefits, and self-fulfillment for the employees as well as value to the community. Value creation can arise from activities in two areas: financial activities and other managerial activities.

Creating value from financial activities focuses mainly on changing the capital structure, mergers and acquisitions, and distributing dividends. This activity is carried out at the level of a firm's management and board of directors.

In this chapter, we focus on the creation of value from nonfinancial activities because they have a significant potential to increase a firm's value and because this subject has been addressed to a lesser extent in practice and in academic research. Such value is created by strategic changes, changing the business or organizational structure, increasing throughput in operations and logistics, improving inventory levels, improving the information systems, and shortening development times.

Changes in cost-accounting and performance measures or improvements in decision-making processes can substantially improve a firm's value. Moreover, as we have seen in previous chapters, the "blind" use of traditional cost accounting and the use of local performance measures can lead to a decrease in the value of firms and organizations.

Sometimes decisions concerning investments and business, organizational, and operational changes are made that do not necessarily contribute to improving the value of the firm. In many cases, this is caused by the *absence of a global perspective and lack of knowledge and an organized method for improving the value of the firm*. As a result, the firm's resources are used ineffectively, its value is not increased sufficiently, management's time is wasted, and its attention is diverted from matters that are important to the firm and which, if properly addressed, could increase its value. In this chapter, we present the subject of firm value and the various methods of assessing it and develop a focused model for creating a link between changes in the various areas of the organization and increasing its value.

Assessing the Value of a Firm

Firm value is a concept commonly used by investors, managers, owners, and boards of directors. Its use is particularly prevalent when a firm is being bought and sold, during mergers, when partners are co-opted, and in dealings with interested parties. Several approaches are used in assessing firm value:

• *Market value:* The value as assessed by the stock market. This immediate assessment is, of course, relevant to traded public firms. However, experience shows that when the level of trade is low, a substantial gap may be created between the "true" value of the firm, as reflected in purchasing transactions and the transfer of control, and its value according to the latest stock market prices reflecting low and insignificant trading.
• *Actual transactions:* The value can be determined by transactions carried out in fact, in raising capital and co-opting partners in

the firm, by exchanging shares, by mergers and acquisitions, or through all of these.

• *Asset value:* The asset value or worth of the firm's equity is the worth of the assets minus the worth of the liabilities.

• *Discounted cash flow:* The basic assumption of discounted cash flows is that the worth of a business is the current value of the discounted cash flows over time. The firm's operational assets and the components of the working capital are needed to attain the cash flows, and their worth to the business is expressed in the discounted cash flow. In analyzing value, the present value of the unleveraged free cash flows is assessed. This amount represents the value of the activities. We must add the value of the "available" assets, which are not required to create cash flows—for example, investments in real estate that are not for purposes of the firm's operations or cash surpluses. From this result, we subtract the worth of the net financial liabilities on the day of the valuation to obtain the worth of the firm to the shareholders. Academically, this method is considered more acceptable and correct. It is suitable for measuring the contribution of management to improving firm value, enabling the measuring of cash flows arising from the activities of the different sectors of the firm and their sources of finance.

The approach of this book in general and of this chapter in particular is to enhance the economic value of a firm, as it is reflected in the cash flow over time. We believe that in the long run, the economic value of a firm will level out at its market value.

The Economic Value-Added Measure

The economic value-added (EVA) metric measures the periodic (for example, annual) increase in shareholders' value. We demonstrate this metric with the aid of a simple numerical example.

There are two firms in the market. Firm A has equity of $600,000 and achieved an end-of-year net operating profit after taxes (NOPAT) of

$100,000. In parallel, firm B has equity of $1 million and achieved a NOPAT of $150,000.

In the example, which of the two firms achieved the better result? The answer is not simple. True, the manager of firm B achieved a higher profit, but he also used a larger amount of capital. We assume, for simplicity, that all investments were made using the equity of the firms and that they did not have any debt.

The EVA measure will give us a satisfactory answer to the above question. First presented by Stewart (1994), it measures the periodic value creation of the firm. Measuring the EVA presents a systematic way that takes into consideration the requested rate of return on a firm's capital. The EVA is expressed in tax-free terms.

Economic value added is defined as the difference between the net operating profit after taxes (before financial costs) and the annual cost of a firm's capital (the equity and the debt used to generate this operating profit).

Economic value added (EVA) = net operating profit after taxes (NOPAT) – weighted average cost of capital (WACC) × invested capital

---

The meaning of the EVA calculation is that an "economic value added" is created for the shareholders only when the operating profit after taxes and before financing costs (NOPAT) is higher than the annual cost of the capital taken for financing the firm's investments (and all in tax-deducted terms, which take into account the tax shelter on the firm's interest expenses). When the NOPAT is smaller than the annual cost of the capital invested in the firm, the shareholders' value is reduced. It should be noted that firms with negative EVA are not necessarily losing firms. They are, rather, firms that do not compensate the owners of capital for their inherent risk and sometimes even show a rate of return that is lower than the rate of return on risk-free assets.

Table 18.1 shows that there is a difference between the ranking of the above firms by other measures and their ranking by EVA. Profit alone does not take into account the capital invested in the firm. The table shows that even though firm A has a higher return on assets, its EVA is lower. A situation is possible in which a firm has a positive NOPAT and a positive net profit but a negative EVA—that is, it diminishes its shareholders' value.

The EVA measure has attracted much managerial attention, and today many firms routinely use it. It can be seen as a measuring tool that determines if the business is earning more than the real cost of the capital invested in it. In other words, EVA is a measuring tool that enables managers, shareholders, and potential investors to examine whether the business creates value or diminishes the value for the shareholders (Stern and Shiely, 2001).

Criticism has been leveled at the use of EVA as the main measure for evaluating the level of performance. For instance, AT&T, which was one of the first to adopt the EVA measure at the beginning of the 1990s, reported after several years of implementing it that it had been forced to add two additional nonfinancial measures

Table 18.1. Return on Assets (ROA) and Economic Value Added (EVA).

	Firm A	Firm B
Assets ($)	600,000	1,000,000
Net operating profit after taxes ($)	100,000	150,000
Return on assets (operating profit) (%)	16.67	15.00
Required profit at a rate of return of 10% net ($)	60,000	100,000
Economic value added (profit after deducting required profit on capital) ($)	40,000	50,000

to it: customers' value added and employees' value added. Following the appointment of a new president in 1997, the firm decided to stop the use of the EVA measure (Horngren, Foster, and Datar, 2000). Nevertheless, we are convinced that despite this criticism, the use of EVA is far preferable to that of any other financial accounting measure proposed to date. Moreover, it should be remembered that a measure is not a substitute for effective management, and management has to examine loopholes that appear in performance measures and close them.

The Value-Focused Management Model

We propose the use of the value-focused management (VFM) model for increasing organizational value. The VFM model helps managers focus on places in which the potential for increasing firm value is greatest, bearing in mind the limited management resources. The model is based on the principles of value-based management, as presented by Copeland, Koller, and Murrin (1996), together with additional elements.

The VFM model boasts the following two dimensions:

- It details the action items required in the field for creating value.

- It focuses managerial attention on the important activities that give the highest value, taking into account an organization's limited resources, particularly the managerial resources that are in short supply.

The stages of implementing the VFM model are as follows:

1. Determine the goal.
2. Determine the performance measures.
3. Identify the value drivers.

4. Decide how to improve the value drivers.

5. Implement and control.

Determine the Goal

The goal of a firm is to increase shareholders' value. This should be clear to all managers and employees. The goal can be sustained over time if at the same time the interests of the employees, the suppliers, the customers, and the community are borne in mind.

Determine the Performance Measures

The performance measures include the financial statements and the global performance measures of the system (see the six measures in Chapter 4). The EVA measure examines the increase in the firm's value periodically.

Identify the Value Drivers

A *value driver* is defined as an important factor that significantly affects the value of the firm, such as increasing sales, increasing throughput, shortening response time, and reducing inventories.

Four approaches are used to identify the relevant cost drivers.

1. *Balance sheet and profit-and-loss statements approach:* Sections of the balance sheet and the profit-and-loss statement are reviewed one at a time to identify potential firm improvement against the ease of carrying out the improvement, using the focusing matrix (described in Chapter 3).

2. *The functional approach, from the bottom up:* The major functions in the organization are reviewed systematically and examined for the existence of relevant value drivers. Such functional areas may include the following:

The organization's strategy

Marketing and sales

Human resources

Information systems and information technology

Finance

Technological innovation

Clinical quality

Service quality

Logistics and purchasing

Operations of wards, labs, and other departments

Cost accounting and measuring

Organizational structure

Risk management

Customer service

The review of the functions is carried out by interviewing the management and the organization's key personnel, touring the premises, perusing the financial and management statements, interviewing customers and suppliers, and comparing with other similar organizations. Attention is then directed to the important value drivers from among those selected, with the help of the focusing matrix. The importance of each value driver is measured according to the incremental value it affords the firm.

3. *The global performance measures approach:* The global performance measures (see Chapter 13) are reviewed one at a time, and the potential increment to the firm's value from improving them is examined.

4. *Identifying the core problems, from the top down:* After collecting the data in stages 1, 2, and 3, the undesirable effects are mapped, and the core problems are identified using the focused current reality tree approach (see Chapter 7).

The relevant value drivers (up to ten) are collected using the above-mentioned four methods. Using the focusing table and the focusing matrix, the potential for each value driver to add to the firm's value and the difficulty of implementation are examined. This process ends with the selection of the value drivers to be used for improving the firm's value.

A detailed implementation plan for improving each of the value drivers is prepared using the innovative managerial techniques described in Parts Two and Three of this book.

Implement and Control

The implementation of the plan and its control are the responsibility of the management.

Strategic Value Drivers

Strategy is the way that the management of an organization takes to reach its goal. An organizational strategy should express the directions of the organization by considering the following questions:

- What are the firm's products and services, and what should be their market positioning?

- What is the market in which the organization is competing?

- What are the organization's core competences, and how can they be preserved?

- What are the weaknesses and vulnerabilities, and how can the organization protect itself from them?

- What is the firm's strategic breakthrough plan?

- What is the organizational policy regarding price and quality of its services and products?

- What is the desired growth rate of the firm?

- What investment level is needed?

- What are the strategic elements that produced sustainable competitive advantage?

- What is the market segmentation and service or product differentiation of the firm's products or services vis-à-vis the competition?

- Where should the firm's constraint be located?

- What should the capital structure of the firm be?

- What should the business and organizational structure of the firm be?

The answers to these questions and others shape the functional strategies in the areas of marketing, sales, finances, technology, information systems, operations, logistics, quality, human resources, and risk management of the firm.

Some of the value drivers that can enhance the value of a health care organization are *strategic value drivers*. The following can be such value drivers:

- Changing the strategy of the organization from a highly varied service provider to a more focused one

- Moving from a nonprofit organization to a for-profit one

- Privatizing a public hospital

- Creating profit centers in public health care organizations

- Decentralizing a health maintenance organization (HMO)

- Adopting a prevention strategy rather than a treatment one

- Changing the organization's attitude to focus on the customer (instead of "treating patients")

Case Study: Queen Medical Center

We now examine a case study for value enhancement in a large not-for-profit hospital.

The Hospital

Queen Medical Center is a fifteen-hundred-bed hospital employing over four thousand workers, including about eight hundred physicians. The hospital has an ED; a surgical division that includes ORs and inpatient wards; a gynecological division with ORs and inpatient wards; and departments of internal medicine, ophthalmology, and all other departments common to a large hospital.

The hospital is considered the leading and best in the area and enjoys reputation and prestige in all areas of operation. It is a university teaching hospital, and its physicians train dozens of medical students and physicians every year. The hospital meets its budget. Its main customers are four large HMOs that provide coverage to the entire regional population. The hospital is known for its technological innovation and its tendency to be a world leader in adopting new diagnostic and therapeutic approaches.

The hospital is professionally managed by a group of physicians with extensive managerial training and experience. The hospital has laboratories and imaging services that are among the best in the world and enjoys a stable workforce with low employee turnover. The hospital is proud of being a technology leader and is open to innovation.

The hospital operates outpatient clinics that serve about 350,000 patients per year. There are 700 annual deliveries and 26,000 operations per year. The ED serves about 111,000 patients per year.

Let us now examine the enhancement potential of the hospital using the VFM approach. As mentioned in the beginning of this chapter, the value of a not-for-profit organization is increased by improving its performance measures vis-à-vis its goal.

Step 1: Determine the Goal

The goal of the hospital is to increase *medical value* by providing high-quality medical service and treatment to as many patients as possible within short response times while maintaining a balanced budget.

Step 2: Determine Performance Measures

The following are the hospital's performance measures:

- Clinical quality measures

- Service quality measures

- Strategic innovation measures

- Throughput

- Response time

- Cash flow

- Annual profit

- Customer satisfaction

- Worker satisfaction

Step 3: Identify the Value Drivers

Different approaches are used to identify the value drivers.

Identify Value Drivers from Relevant Sections in the Hospital's Financial Statements

There is high profitability in the outpatient clinics. Thus, analyzing the potential of the outpatient clinic, a potential value driver could be to increase the outpatient clinics' throughput.

Use a Bottom-Up Approach to Identify Functional Value Drivers

To be able to identify the functional value drivers for the hospital, let us review the functional area one by one:

- *Hospital strategy:* The hospital provides an array of services and is considered the best in its region. The hospital strategy is based on providing the best clinical service, using advanced technologies, and attracting renowned specialists to improve the relevant quality. The hospital management has a business orientation and finances some of its expenses by building support services on the hospital campus: a hotel for patients' families, restaurants, and parking lots. The hospital is also investing in advanced technologies and is a partner in various start-up companies. An analysis of the hospital's strengths, weaknesses, opportunities, and threats is presented in Table 18.2.

- *Marketing, sales, and business development:* These are performed extremely well.

- *Human resources:* The employees are dedicated, but there is a sense of alienation between management and employees. Most of the department heads are superb professionals in their specialty, but they lack management vision and training. The physicians have an inherent conflict between their own interest (private practice) and the hospital goal.

- *Information technology:* The hospital has good management information systems that enable it to exercise control over budgets and timetables. Using advanced technologies, the hospital is running a pilot of implementing an electronic record.

- *Finance:* The hospital is financially sound.

- *Emergency department:* During day hours, the ED is managed professionally, and patients receive quality treatment both clinically and from a service perspective. In the afternoon and evening hours, the situation is different, with the formation of long queues. The average wait is four hours. There is no systematic and structured

Table 18.2. Analysis of Queen Medical Center's Strengths, Weaknesses, Opportunities, and Threats.

Strengths	Weaknesses
A variety of services	High managerial complexity
Excellent reputation	Management level of wards not sufficient
High clinical level	
Innovative and dynamic management	Worker dissatisfaction
	Unstructured processes in the wards
Professional management and business orientation	
	Local and sectoral optimization
High technological capability	

Opportunities	Threats
Development of business ventures of services in the hospital	Competitors may close the clinical and technological gap
Purchase of new technologies and techniques	Excess capacity in other hospitals in the region may lead to a price war
Development of new technologies and techniques	Tight contracts with the main customer

scheduling and prioritization. The ED relations with the hospital (on-call and specialty consultants) are not congruent with the load. During the evening and night hours, there is a severe shortage of specialists in emergency medicine and general and orthopedic surgeons. There is great potential to reduce the long waits.

• *Operating rooms:* The clinical quality of the surgical procedures is high, and the technological know-how is advanced. There is an obvious segmentation (surgeons, anesthetists, and surgical nurses). There are idle times in the ORs, and the anesthetists are the bottleneck. Too many people are involved in managing the ORs (head surgical nurse, head of the division of surgery, and head of the anesthetics department). Management is insufficiently integrated, and the scheduling of operations does not meet the needs. The bottlenecks are not sufficiently utilized, and the logistics department is not involved enough.

• *Outpatient clinics:* The outpatient clinics serve about 350,000 patients annually. There is potential to increase this number by improving efficiency and effectiveness and enhancing marketing.

• *Management of other wards in the hospital:* Undoubtedly, there is room for improvement in other departments in the hospital. The main concern and the potential value driver is the managerial quality of the management team. During the hospital evaluation process, it was decided to focus on the departments with the highest potential for enhancement. At this stage, management will not direct improvements in the other wards because it seems that the potential is not as large as in the ED, the ORs, and other places. Any department head wishing to make improvements in his or her department, at his or her initiative, will receive management support and appropriate budgets.

• *Technology and innovation:* Queen Medical Center is one of the world leaders in technological innovation, both in equipment and treatment.

• *Quality:* Clinical quality is measured systematically and meets world standards. Service quality is excellent in some departments, and there is room for improvement in others.

• *Logistics and purchasing:* The logistics are complex because of the large variety of services provided in the hospital. Logistical problems in the OR cause occasional delays due to shortages in some items. There is a need to shift toward standardizing OR equipment and careful preparation of kits there. Purchasing costs are relatively high, and there is potential for price and inventory reduction.

• *Pricing and costing:* Most decisions are made by management using a global view, taking resource capacity and marginal profitability into consideration. The approach by midlevel management is based on traditional cost accounting.

- *Organizational structure:* The organizational structure is based on divisions that consist of the various departments. The current structure is somewhat problematic, but management decided to first deal with the "low-hanging fruit" that will bring about immediate improvement. Only later will management discuss changing the organizational structure, which is difficult to do and whose contribution is questionable.

- *Risk management:* A separate department manages risk in a professional manner.

- *Customer service:* A customer service department handles customer complaints and tries to identify process improvements.

As a result of this summary and with the use of the focusing matrix, the following potential value drivers were identified:

- Reduce waits in the ED.

- Increase throughput in the ORs.

- Increase throughput in the outpatient clinics.

- Improve logistics and purchasing.

Identify Value Drivers Using Global Performance Measures

A review of the various performance measures identified the following potential value drivers:

- Establish due date performance in the ORs and adhere to it.

- Reduce response time in the ED.

- Increase throughput in the ORs.

Examine a Top-Down Approach to Value Drivers

At first, the following relevant undesirable effects for the hospital were identified:

- Medical value is not sufficient: the hospital does not fulfill its potential

- Insufficient revenues

- Critical resources are not fully utilized

- Sense of workforce shortage

- High level of complexity

- Insufficient managerial level in some departments

- Complicated organizational structure

- The outpatient clinics do not meet their potential

- ORs are not fully utilized

- Local and segmented optimization

- Alienation between management and workers

- Processes are not sufficiently structured

- Conflict of interest between the personal welfare of physicians and the welfare of the hospital

- Long waits in the ED

The focused current reality for the hospital, which contains the above-named undesirable effects, is presented in Figure 18.1. The tree facilitates the identification of the core problems of the hospital. The core problems are potential value drivers. Thus, dealing with the core problems will enhance the value of the hospital.

Choose the Relevant Value Drivers

After reviewing the list of potential value drivers, management decided to focus on the following drivers:

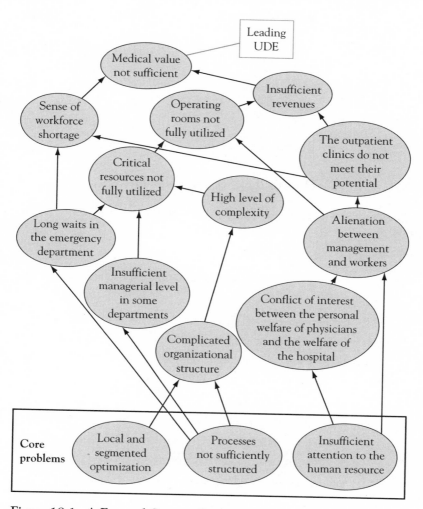

Figure 18.1. A Focused Current Reality Tree for Queen Medical Center.

- Increase OR throughput.

- Reduce waits in the ED.

- Increase the throughput in the outpatient clinics.

- Reduce purchasing costs.

- Cultivate the human resource.

Step 4: Decide How to Improve the Value Drivers

Decisions to improve the value drivers are detailed below.

A. *Increase OR Throughput*

The OR's throughput will be increased by taking the following steps:

- *Exploit the constraint:* The constraint (bottleneck) is the anesthetists' time. In various measurements that were taken, it was determined that the ORs are utilized only 60 percent of the time, mainly due to inefficient time of the anesthetists.

Operations start late. Even though all the resources are available at 8:00 A.M., the first operation does not begin before 8:30 A.M. or even 8:45 A.M. Measuring the start time of surgery and making sure that the first one starts early may help solve most of this problem.

Operations end early. The shift ends at 4:00 P.M., so surgeons avoid starting long operations in the afternoon. A change in the OR scheduling where the long operations are scheduled at the beginning of the day and the short ones at the end may solve this problem.

Setup times between operations are long. Shortening the various steps of entering the patient into the OR, administering initial anesthesia, immediate removal to recovery, and rapid cleaning can all contribute to increasing anesthetists' and OR utilization.

Operations are canceled because of incomplete kits.

- *Elevate the constraint:* Analyzing the labor content of the anesthetists revealed that because the hospital is a teaching hospital, the number of residents is relatively large in comparison with other hospitals in general and with university hospitals in particular. Reducing the number of residents can help increase OR throughput.
- *Improve scheduling:* Scheduling patients using the drum-buffer-rope approach (see Chapter 5) can contribute to constraint exploitation. Some of the scheduling can be done by the wards and some through central scheduling and appointments.
- *Integrate OR management:* In the OR, there are too many managers (head nurse, head of anesthesia, and head of surgical division, who is in charge of scheduling). Appointing a "plant manager" to the OR complex and making that person in charge of the site, the scheduling, and the logistics may help solve the problem.
- *Incorporate logistics:* Preparing kits ahead of time and introducing new processes of team work can help increase the number of operations and their quality.

All the above steps can increase the number of operations by 20 percent in six months with the current mix of operations. (Note that the existing mix of operations can be changed, at least in part, but management has decided not to do so because of the public nature of the hospital.)

All of the above activities can be done with minimal investment. The difficulty of performing these steps is moderate: it is rather easy to exploit the constraints, but the need to coordinate several departments that are not subordinated to one another makes the task more difficult.

To get a better feel for the importance of increasing OR throughput, let us examine this through profitability. The current expense structure of the surgical division is as follows:

Sales	$100
Variable costs	10
Fixed costs	85
Profit	$ 5

After increasing throughput by 15 percent with the same resources, the picture is as follows:

Sales	$115.00
Variable costs	11.50
Fixed costs	85.00
Profit	$ 18.50

Thus, the potential for enhancement exceeds 300 percent! Assuming that the profits from the increased throughput are mostly invested in the hospital (with the minority used to reward physicians or as dividends for the government who owns the hospital), this improvement withstands any standard of the objective function of the hospital. Hence, this value driver will be rated 5 on the importance scale (very important).

B. *Reduce Waiting Times in the ED*

Waiting times in the ED will be reduced by the following steps:

• *Improving scheduling, ordering, and follow-up*: The improvement approach will be through a proactive and dynamic buffer management. This method is based on first identifying the causes of the waits. Using the Pareto approach, the major causes are identified as follows:

- Waiting for x-ray films and other imaging services
- Waiting for a surgical consultant
- Waiting for the discharge letter

A team consisting of the ED chief and representatives of hospital management can help resolve these problems.

As a second step, management will define the maximal accepted wait for 95 percent of patients (for example, four hours). Every patient will have his or her arrival time recorded, and after the first hour, follow-up will be conducted by three buffer zones ("traffic lights"):

Green zone: ED time between zero and two hours. In this zone, only the patient's status will be recorded.

Yellow zone: ED time of two to three hours. In this zone, data will be collected on the reasons for delay.

Red zone: waiting time of three to four hours. In this zone, the supervising nurse initiates an expediting process and records data on the cause of the delay.

The hospital management will convene with the ED management once a week, will use a Pareto diagram or focusing matrix of the reasons for delays, and will take corrective actions. This approach yields three outcomes:

1. Order and priorities in managing ED time are introduced.
2. Actions are expedited when needed.
3. The real problems are identified, using a global perspective, and corrective actions taken.

- *Change the organizational structure of the ED:* The idea is to form autonomous units of emergency medicine specialists, thus reducing the dependence on outside consultants. This can be done by recruiting nonoperating general and orthopedic surgeons (for example, retired from operating). Hospital management decided that this step would be considered six months after implementing the previous step. The ease of implementing this step was assessed at 4, and its importance for value enhancement at 5.

C. Increase Outpatient Clinic Throughput

Outpatient clinic throughput will be increased by negotiating with the major customers (the four HMOs), exploiting the competitive advantage of high clinical quality, excellent reputation, fast response times, and attractive prices. These actions can increase outpatient clinic throughput by 5 percent. The ease of implementing this step was determined to be 4, and its importance, 4.

D. Reduce Purchasing Costs

Purchasing costs will be reduced by classifying suppliers into A, B, and C groups and focusing on group A suppliers. Seven suppliers were identified, accounting for 65 percent of purchases. In parallel, the purchased items were classified, and seventy-five items were found to account for 85 percent of purchasing costs.

By focusing on these items and suppliers, negotiating with the suppliers better, and carefully analyzing the needed quantities, it is possible to achieve a 5 percent savings in purchasing costs. The ease of implementation was assessed at 4 and its importance at 5.

E. Deal with the Human Resource

The alienation felt by the workers from management ("us versus them") caused mistrust and frustration. This requires immediate attention. The human resource will be dealt with at the following several levels:

- The hospital CEO and a team of top management will meet with *all* employees in the hospital in departmental and divisional meetings.

- Team-forging activities will be initiated for the entire hospital, in addition to activities in each department.

- A permanent process will be created that will monitor workers' feelings and provide a forum for expressing their comments on a monthly basis.

- Some of the CEO's time will be allocated to random interviews with employees and attempts to resolve some of the problems that cause alienation.

The above five value drivers are presented in the focusing table given in Table 18.3. In addition, we can map the improvement potential using the focusing matrix (easy-important) given in Figure 18.2.

The Improvement Implementing Process

Management decided to start working on value drivers A, B, and E: increase OR throughput, reduce ED waiting times, and deal with the human resource. Although difficult to deal with (see Figure

Table 18.3. Focusing Table for Queen Medical Center Value Drivers.

Designation	Value Driver	Importance[a]	Ease of Implementing[b]
A	Increase OR throughput	5	3
B	Reduce waiting times in the ED	5	4
C	Increase outpatient clinic throughput	4	4
D	Reduce purchasing costs	5	4
E	Deal with the human resource	4	2

[a]Scale is 1 (unimportant) to 5 (important).
[b]Scale is 1 (very difficut) to 5 (very easy).

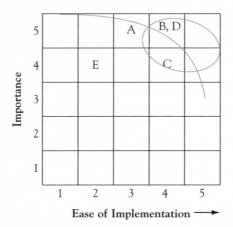

Figure 18.2. Focusing Matrix for Value Enhancement at Queen Medical Center, Based on Table 18.3.

18.2), management has considered the human aspect to be important and has decided to deal with it as soon as possible. The other value drivers will be dealt with at a later stage because currently management time that can be devoted to the change process is insufficient, as is the organizational ability to absorb too many changes in a short time. These steps will be postponed to a later stage that will begin in about six months.

Chapter Summary

Enhancing an organization's value is the goal of its managers. In this chapter, we presented a practical approach to increase the value of the firm, especially through dealing with managerial issues and measuring the contribution to the value of the firm. The VFM method, presented in this chapter, enables managers to examine where they should devote their time and energy and in which areas the contribution will be marginally small. The method can be used in both for-profit and not-for-profit organizations.

Part IV

Summary

19

Case Study

The Emergency Department at Guard Mountain Hospital

Objective

- Learn through a case study how to integrate and implement the simple methods of this book

Background

The emergency department (ED) of Guard Mountain Hospital (GMH) serves a population of 300,000 people. GMH is a teaching hospital and is considered the largest and best medical center in the region. It has 1,500 beds and employs more than 800 physicians and about 1,800 nursing staff.

The ED sees over 100,000 people annually, a third of whom are admitted to the hospital while the others are discharged to their home or to the community for follow-up. The staff consists of fifteen physicians trained in emergency medicine and about fifty nurses. The head of the ED is a board-certified emergency medicine specialist with over twenty years' experience. A head nurse oversees the nursing staff.

The head of the ED, together with the hospital director, has decided to embark on a continuous improvement process with the following goals:

- Improve the clinical quality provided by the ED.

- Shorten the response times and patients' waits.

- Improve the quality of service given to the ED patients.

The Improvement Process

A short assessment was conducted to find the core problems and the most effective value drivers. This was mainly done to have an independent opinion on the implementation process that will be led by the ED personnel and to adapt the executive workshop to the special environment of the ED.

The senior staff of the ED attended a three-day executive workshop to determine the department's goals and to learn the focused management approach. Together they drafted an implementation plan. This workshop was preceded by a similar workshop attended by hospital management. This resulted in choosing the ED and operating rooms (ORs) as the ones to focus system improvement on. During the workshop, the following concepts were discussed, and the participants have suggested action items for implementation.

Managing the System's Constraints

To manage the system's constraints, the team first focused on the goal of the ED and its performance measures. It was then possible to identify, exploit, subordinate, and relieve the constraints.

It was decided that the goal of the ED was to provide maximal clinical quality and to treat all patients within a minimal time. The following performance measures, some of which were already measured, were outlined by the group:

- *Throughput:* Number of patients, percentage hospitalized, percentage discharged home.

- *Operating expenses:* Personnel costs, number of ED physicians, number of ED nurses, number of ED ancillary staff.

- *Work in process:* The amount of work in process (WIP) was defined as the average number of patients in the ED. The WIP should be measured twice daily, during day hours (off-peak) and during evening hours (peak).

- *Response time:* The response time was measured from the time of entry into the ED until the time the patient was discharged home or the time the patient was physically admitted to one of the hospital wards. The ED director preferred measuring the median time rather than the average time because this measure better reflects the actual nature of the system.

- *Quality:* The following clinical quality measures were decided on:

  - Percentage of discharged patients who returned to the ED within twenty-four hours

  - Percentage of patients leaving the premises without completing the treatment (against medical advice)

  - Quality of clinical diagnosis of hospitalized patients: it was decided to consider several common diagnoses and randomly check the diagnosis after hospitalization compared with that in the ED.

- *Due date performance:* A standard of 2.5 hours was chosen as the mode time spent in the ED. The percentage of patients meeting this standard was used as one of the performance measures.

Identifying the Constraints

During peak hours—Monday mornings and every evening starting at 6:00 P.M.—there is a *resource constraint,* and the bottleneck is experienced emergency physicians. There is certainly a market constraint during Tuesday through Friday every morning from 8:00 A.M. to about 10:00 A.M. In addition, several *dummy constraints* have been identified:

- Lack of personnel for transporting patients and equipment

- Lack of enough automatic blood pressure monitors

- Missing electrocardiograph machines

- Lack of such basics as wheelchairs or stepping stools

- Lack of lab pneumatic tubes

Policy constraints have been identified as well:

- Several lab tests are not performed twenty-four hours per day.

- There is lack of synchronization of the starting times between physicians and nurses.

- In the morning hours, there is an excess capacity of emergency physicians whereas in the afternoons they are in short supply.

Exploiting the Constraints

It turns out that the ED physicians are wasting 30 percent of their time, for the following reasons. First of all, there are many "mental setups" because of the long stay of patients in the ED, waiting for admission to the hospital, expert consultants, lab results, imaging results, and conveyance.

The ED physicians also perform many tasks that are beyond the core of their activity, including drawing blood, applying casts, approving decisions regarding referral of patients by nurses for imaging or other tests, suturing simple wounds, as well as communicating with the wards and arguing about hospitalization authority and communicating with family members who are pressuring to speed up the process.

It also seems that experienced ED physicians do not use excess testing, and they have proposed several improvements for the professional competency of the physicians and nurses.

Subordinating to the Constraint

The teams that were coordinated during the workshop examined the situation and found that subordination to the ED physicians was adequately done.

Relieving the Constraint (Offloading)

The workshop teams suggested that nurses should assume responsibility for some of the tasks performed by the ED physicians in the following ways:

- Give the nursing staff more authority (to refer patients for imaging and other tests).

- Transfer some of the nurses' duties to technicians and ancillary personnel.

- Authorize the nurses to perform some of the medical procedures.

- Authorize a nurse or casting person to perform some of the suturing and to apply casts.

Examining the Adverse Effects of WIP

The staff has examined the drawbacks of the WIP of patients and found the following consequences:

- The long waits result in diminished clinical quality.

- The longer presence of patients and their family members engages the staff in time-consuming discussions about the long stay and occasionally results in violence against staff members.

- The long waits cause a delay in detecting high-risk patients.

- Control over services performed outside the ED (imaging, consultants) is not effective because of the large number of patients waiting for these services.

- Because of the long waiting times and the large number of WIP patients, follow-up of tests results is diminished.

- The ED physicians engage in bad multitasking.

Solutions to Reducing WIP

The ED staff decided on the following actions to reduce WIP:

- *Managing bottlenecks:* There will be a thorough analysis of the possibilities to exploit, subordinate to, and relieve the ED physicians that are the bottleneck in the system.
- *Strategic gating:* It turns out that 10 percent of patients passing through the ED do not need its medical services and are there because of a hospital admission policy that requires all admissions to use that route. These include patients entering for some elective surgeries, patients requiring nursing, and so forth. The ED staff wants to investigate channels for directly admitting such patients or establishing a separate channel through the ED at nonpeak hours. This problem is not significant and will be dealt with later.
- *Tactical gating:* An experienced nurse currently performs triage. The staff feels that the triage process can be improved along the following lines:

- Give the triage nurse wider authority to order lab and imaging tests.

- Expand the complete kit that the triage nurse gives the ED staff to include a synopsis of the patient from the health maintenance organization (something that can be done using the existing information systems).

- Allow just one accompanying person per patient (in most cases).

- *Working with small batches:* The recommendation was made to immediately dispatch of every test and to notify the expert consultant on every waiting patient. It is important to convince the staff that accumulating patients before summoning an expert increases the WIP, along with all its undesirable effects, especially long response times.

- *Building the "traffic lights" system:* The hospital adopted the theory of constraints approach and modified the buffer management technique to reduce waiting times by using a traffic light approach. According to this approach, the standard allowed waiting time of 2.5 hours is divided into three parts, as seen in Figure 19.1. Patients in the yellow zone are actively managed to avoid their moving into the red zone. Patients in the red zone are expedited through the remaining steps in the system, and the causes for their waiting are

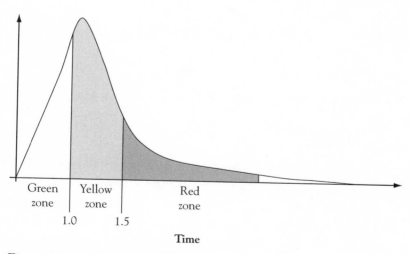

Figure 19.1. The Traffic Light Zones.

monitored. A major step in the improved process is the "traffic light meetings." A multidisciplinary management team should meet for thirty minutes every week to identify the major causes of delay and develop an implementation plan to quickly eradicate these causes and escalate systemwide policy issues.

• *Reducing bad multitasking:* The ED staff feels that awareness of bad multitasking will automatically reduce it.

• *Peak management:* There is a need to synchronize the work schedule of the ED physicians and nurses with the peak demand. For example, on Tuesdays through Fridays, demand is low before 10 A.M. Thus, it was suggested that physicians have a later start to their workday, which will extend into the late afternoon, when demand is higher. It was also suggested that during peak hours, priority should be given to the lab and to transportation of patients and that during the slow ED morning hours, priority should be shifted to the wards where morning rounds are taking place.

• *Breaking dummy constraints:* The ED nurses were required to answer phone inquiries about the hospital during the night shift. These calls must be handled by other personnel.

• *The complete kit concept:* The workshop revealed that there are several possibilities for improvement in several kit types:

• Protocols for patient management

• A complete kit for admission (in-kit and out-kit)

• A complete kit for consultants (in-kit and out-kit)

The ED staff realized that working with incomplete in-kits and out-kits causes many problems. An incomplete in-kit resulted in a waste of time and resources, duplication of work and tests, possible errors in diagnosis and treatment, and a decline in motivation. Likewise, an incomplete out-kit resulted in inadequate treatment, damage to the ED's reputation and prestige, and rework due to questions and inquiries.

The ED team has decided to design and update forms and protocols of complete kits for the most frequently performed procedures and treatments.

Focused Current Reality Tree

Participants in the workshop drew a focused current reality tree and reached the conclusion presented in Figure 19.2.

Action Items

At the end of the workshop, the participants summarized the proposed action items using the focusing table and the focusing matrix shown in Table 19.1 and Figure 19.3, respectively.

Creation of Teams

At the conclusion of the workshop, it was decided to establish seven teams to deal with the following topics:

1. Preparing kits and guidelines
2. Reducing response times vis-à-vis the labs
3. Improving information systems and building a traffic light system
4. Maintenance and equipment
5. Change in management policy
6. Triage: improvement and interdepartmental cross-training
7. Exploiting and managing bottlenecks

A detailed mission for each team is shown in Table 19.2.

Chapter Summary

This chapter provided an in-depth analysis of a real-world situation and detailed the various steps to guide such an evaluation.

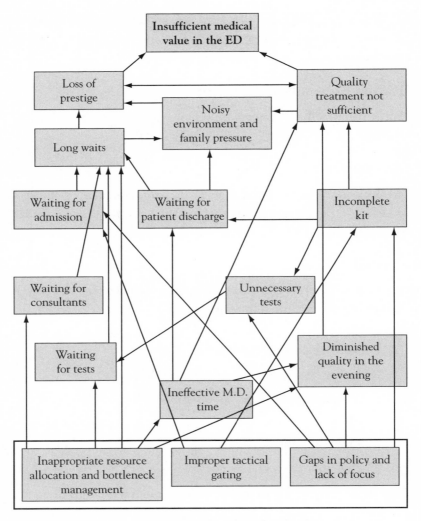

Figure 19.2. Focused Current Reality Tree for the ED.

Table 19.1. Focusing Table for the ED Action Items.

Number	Activity	Importance[a]	Ease of Implementing[b]
1	Reducing response times vis-à-vis the labs	4	4
2	Improving equipment and maintenance	3	4
3	Improving the triage process	5	4
4	Writing guidelines and implementing the complete kit concept	5	4
5	Implementing traffic light control	5	5
6	Exploiting and offloading bottlenecks	4	4
7	Changing hospital policy on synchronizing resources	4	2

[a]Scale is 1 (unimportant) to 5 (important).
[b]Scale is 1 (very difficult) to 5 (very easy).

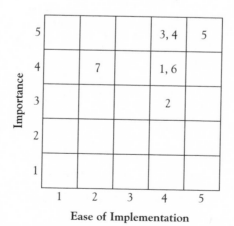

Figure 19.3. Focusing Matrix for the ED Action Items, Based on Table 19.1.

Table 19.2. Action Items for Teamwork.

Topic	Items for Action
Reducing response times vis-à-vis the labs	Labs: Until 10:00 A.M., will be subordinated to wards; after that, subordinated to the ED
	Labs are not accessible twenty-four hours a day; prepare kits for troponin testing or testing instrument that will be permanently in the ED
	Lab test pneumatic tubes leave the lab once every few hours, with a messenger taking them to a centralized depot, creating a shortage of tubes in the ED; increase frequency of collecting tubes to avoid this dummy constraint
Equipment and maintenance	Dummy constraint: a maintenance person dedicated to the ED is needed, or at least for the floor, who will perform routine maintenance every morning and will handle malfunctions in the ED.
	Dummy constraint: shortage of wheelchairs
	Purchase more simple equipment (intravenous stands, blood pressure monitors) to increase their availability
	Perform better preventive maintenance to equipment that is susceptible to malfunctions
Triage	Assign a control clerk at the triage station
	Focus cross-training of an additional team for triage work
Guidelines and complete kits	Define complete kits (in-kit and out-kit) for consultants and for treatment
	Update guidelines (treatment, diagnostic, triage, holding)
	Define guidelines for referrals to such tests as computed tomographic scans

Table 19.2. Action Items for Teamwork.

Topic	Items for Action
	Improve the complicated referral form for patients to wards
	Determine a minimal information kit that will accompany patients to the wards
Information systems and traffic light control	Measurement: waiting times for consultants and waiting times for hospital wards, in addition to measurements in the ED
	Prepare a traffic light system
	Prepare an electronic bulletin board to display information to the staff (waiting times for consultants and the labs, number of people waiting at each stage, and the like) and a directional board for patients
Bottleneck management and offloading	Flexibly schedule the entire staff, including physicians, to peak times
	Delegate more authority to nurses (as was done with imaging) and train all nurses to draw blood, stitch wounds, and so forth
	Offload the night phone calls to clerks
	A lab technician can offload from nurses obtaining blood tests
	Every section should have volunteers or other low-paid staff to relieve the nurses of simple tasks such as providing patients with tea or blankets or changing bedding
	Every recumbent patient can and should have one accompanying person; this can be done via a sticker system where every patient receives one sticker for himself or herself and one for an escort, and only people with stickers can enter the ED

Table 19.2. Action Items for Teamwork, *continued.*

Topic	Items for Action
	Distribute brochures about the ED process to every patient, and show an explanatory film in the waiting area
Change in hospital policy	Use an internal medicine physician during morning hours in exchange for two ED physicians in the evening
	Exercise admission privileges for ED physicians

20

Our Managerial Credo

It is difficult to determine what is right and not right in management and which management style is best. In a world of uncertainties in markets, technology, and politics, it is important to adapt trade conditions, management methods, and tools to the changing situations. However, we must design a managerial concept that will help increase competitiveness, enhance a firm's value for its owners, and improve the performance measures of the organization.

The Managerial Frame of Mind

In this chapter, we lay out the managerial frame of mind that we feel is the most suitable one for the twenty-first century, with focus on health care organizations.

"The World Is Simpler Than It Seems"

The health care world is complex and complicated. It is affected by dozens, perhaps even hundreds, of factors. It is filled with uncertainty in demand for services, technology, and politics. The various management functions are permanent conflicts (best possible care versus budget constraints). Life cycles of services and products are becoming shorter and shorter. New technologies appear almost daily, and competition puts pressures on all departments in an organization.

As we have shown several times in this book, viewing this world through a different prism makes us realize that this world is simpler than it seems. The approach to simplicity is *focus*. Things seem simpler through focused eyes. For example:

- *Focusing on core problems:* Any health care organization faces a multitude of problems. Trying to solve them one by one will take up all a manager's time and will probably not yield the desired results because this approach treats only the symptoms rather than the problems themselves. Every organization has only a small number of core problems, and focusing on them simplifies matters. Solving (even partially) these core problems relieves most of the symptoms and problems of the organization.
- *Focusing on the system's constraints:* A system has many resources that contribute to its complexity. However, if we focus on the relatively few true system constraints, things become clearer and simpler.
- *Focusing on type A Pareto items:* A health care organization has many failures and quality problems, many suppliers and service providers, a large variety of services and products, a varied array of customers, various raw materials and components, and many performance requirements in every service—indeed, a complicated and complex world. However, if we focus on the few and important type A items, the world will be simpler.
- *Focusing on the "critical path" or the "critical chain":* A typical project in a health care organization consists of hundreds of activities. Careful control and monitoring of many activities concurrently make management complex and complicated. Focusing on the critical path or the critical chain, which contains only a limited number of activities, can greatly simplify the project management.
- *Focusing on key points:* Most processes are complex and complicated. They usually have many stages that add to the complexity, especially if they cross various departments of the organization. Focusing on key points such as *gating* at the beginning of the process

generates fewer control points, which require less effort to handle. Other key points like *buffer management* make the issues simpler and more controllable.

- *Focusing on uncertainty:* Processes in clinical medicine and health care are complex and complicated. Focusing on the factors that contribute most to the uncertainty simplifies the picture and focuses attention on the essential.

All Organizations Are "Sick"

Even though we are focusing on the health care industry, we believe there does not exist a "healthy" organization. This is true for all sectors, not just health care. Organizations operate at only 10 to 20 percent of their potential value or performance. On the one hand, this is a rather dismal situation, but on the other hand, it presents opportunities for dramatic improvements.

A situation where a system operates at low effectiveness and utilization is not rare. This is analogous to engineering or thermodynamics where many engines, for example, operate at single-digit utilization! An organization is a collection of people, resources, and tools that are working to provide some need or have gathered to achieve some goal. The low organizational effectiveness stems from several reasons inherent in the mere existence of the organization and its processes:

- Inherent conflicts

- The goals of the individual and the goals of the organization

- Internal and external uncertainty

- Technological innovation

- Ongoing competition

- The "garbage plant" of the organization

Inherent Conflicts

The *inherent conflicts* in an organization emerge from the ways that the different functions of the organization operate. It would be nice if this friction could be a constructive one, but it usually is not, leading to a reduction of performance. An example is the *development-marketing conflict*: Marketing wants to develop for every customer a unique service with features as close as possible to tailor-made. The development office wants to generate unique leading-edge technology services or products, ones that are also fun to develop.

There is also the *development-production conflict*: The production department prefers to produce one product over time. The development department wants to develop many products and prototypes with short life cycles. These conflicts and others create tension between people and the organization and friction that reduces performance.

The inherent conflicts in an organization also manifest themselves in incomplete measurement of various functions. It is difficult to find local performance measures that will each be congruent with the organization's goals. Thus, there is a gap between the local performance measures (of the medical director of the ward, head nurse, project manager, head of an area, operations manager, marketing director, and so forth) and the performance measure of the whole organization. This gap, known as the *performance measures' gap*, causes deviation from the desired performance of the organization. After all, every system is a subsystem of a broader system, and optimization of a smaller system is liable to be suboptimization of a larger one.

The Goals of the Individual Versus the Goals of the Organization

In the ideal setting, the goals of the individual coincide with those of the organization. The individual usually has goals of self-fulfillment, depending on his or her personality. The organization consists of tens, hundreds, or even thousands of individuals who are in daily contact with management and with one another. Lack of communication and conflicting objectives may lead to low effectiveness of operation.

External and Internal Uncertainty

External and internal uncertainty is a critical factor in reducing organizational effectiveness. External sources of uncertainty include demand, regulation, competition, legislation, politics, quantities and prices of outputs, costs and availability of inputs, and the like. Internal sources of uncertainty include failures in computing services; production failures; quality problems; worker absenteeism; processing time of information, services, and products; and technological uncertainty. All these inhibit organizational effectiveness.

Technological Innovation

Technological innovation accelerates competition and leads to a reduction of the life cycle of every technological system. By the time a technology has been diffused into an organization, it already needs to be improved, changed, or replaced altogether. Before an organization has settled down to providing a service or producing a product, it needs to consider designing a new one. Technological innovation occasionally forces an organization to provide incomplete services or market products that require extensive support and maintenance.

Ongoing Competition

Ongoing competition forces an organization to operate less effectively than had it been a monopoly.

The "Garbage Plant" of the Organization

All the above, and other issues, combine to create a considerable garbage plant. This is the collection of all the activities in the organization that do not add value to the organization in general and particularly to the customers, the products or services, and the processes. It is estimated at dozens of percentages of labor hours and the costs of materials and other inputs. The garbage plant expresses itself in defects that need repairing, mistakes that need correcting, system integration that may last from days to weeks, many unnecessary development cycles, the need to apologize to customers, hours of meetings and discussions to figure out what went wrong and why, and other types of waste like unnecessary inventory, unnecessary conveyance, unneeded activities, and repeat performances.

It is, thus, not surprising that organizations work at only 10 to 20 percent of their potential. How do such organizations survive? The competitors probably have similar problems. The logical conclusion is that improvements in an organization can create a competitive edge, and these improvements can be achieved, among others, by focusing, as was discussed throughout this book.

Taking a Global View

Viewing the system as a whole is just part of the managerial outlook. Every worker and manager must view the whole system from the perspective of top management and take a global view over time. Global vision reduces the phenomenon of suboptimization, where optimizing a subsystem with an objective function that may be different from that of the whole organization reduces the value of the organization.

Managerial Maturity

As we have seen, organizations suffer from a lack of resources, especially in the permanent bottlenecks. Managerial maturity is needed to understand this phenomenon and to manage resources properly. Managerial maturity means that there is a need to knowingly *forgo* tasks, projects, products, services, and customers to be able to focus efforts. For example, a health maintenance organization (HMO) wishes to develop four new services, each one with a potential of being a breakthrough in the health care market. However, development resources are limited and are sufficient for the development of only two services. Management has to decide to forgo the development of two of the services and focus on the two that have the highest potential for enhancing value for the HMO. The dilemma is serious because of the underlying uncertainty: maybe one of the forgone services would be the one that would catapult the HMO beyond its competitors. Managerial maturity is the ability to make brave decisions in the face of uncertainty when it is clear that there is always the possibility of an error in judgment. However, the decision should be made with the *best information* available to the decision makers at the *time of decision*.

Human Resources

All managers must devote much of their time to manage their human resources to extract the potential of the organization. The human resource has the highest potential for improvement on the one hand and the highest variability on the other. Hence, there is a need to devote special managerial attention both for extracting the potential and for realizing the variation among the different people in the organization.

The Satisficer Principle

Nobel laureate H. A. Simon recognized back in the 1960s one of the major managerial problems that stands in the way of decision makers: managers tend to behave as optimizers. An optimizer is one who aspires to reach the best possible decision, regardless of time-frame considerations. There is no doubt that leaning toward being an optimizer will lead to better decisions, but the decision may take way too long. In a dynamic world with frequent changes and where time to market is critical, the world of the optimizers is becoming extinct. In the health care industry, this is summarized in the statement, "Until the doctors decide, the patient will die."

Simon proposes to behave as a satisficer and to make *satisfactory* decisions: establish a reasonable level of aspiration that must be achieved and that leads to a substantial improvement in performance. With the satisficer approach, there is no objective of maximizing or minimizing a performance measure but, rather, of achieving a predetermined satisfactory aspiration level. The objective of modern management is not to find the ideal solution to a problem or the organization but, rather, to achieve significant improvement.

Using Performance Measures

People and systems behave according to how they are measured. "Tell me how you behave, and I will tell you how you are being measured." Choosing and implementing appropriate performance measures will greatly enhance the value of the firm.

Simple Tools

Modern management approaches are based on simplicity and common sense. Experience shows that "what is not simple simply will not be."

The 85-15 Rule: Importance of Process

The modern manager must monitor processes and improve them. The 85-15 rule states that 85 percent of problems resulting from the *process* are under management's responsibility. Only 15 percent of problems are under the responsibility of the employees. Thus, focus should be aimed at improving the process.

The "Ten Times" Rule

A failure that is detected at a particular stage of the process will cause one-tenth the damage occurring if the failure is detected at the next stage. As a result, we must focus on the early stages of the process.

Differentiation

The modern managerial outlook stresses differentiation: differential policy for different cases and different managerial situations.

Implementing Focused Management Methods in a Health Care Organization

In the process of improving organizational value, three questions must be addressed (Goldratt, 1990):

- What should be changed?

- What should it be changed to?

- How should the change be made?

What Should Be Changed?

The goal is to enhance the value of a firm or improve performance in not-for-profit organizations. We will exploit the value drivers to enhance the value of the organization on the one hand and deal with the *value inhibitors* (policy constraints, dummy constraints, weaknesses and threats) on the other. The idea is to focus on a small number of factors that we will try to improve. It is simply impossible to properly focus on too many issues simultaneously.

What Should It Be Changed To?

We will want to utilize the value drivers and enhance the value of the firm over time.

How Should the Change Be Made?

How to make the change is the key question. The principles discussed in this book seem simple, but it takes time to fully implement them in an organization. This is a result of the need to change the minds of many people in the organization and to create a work environment that is open to new ideas and their implementation.

The Process of Change

The process of change has several stages, which are discussed below.

Business Diagnosis

The diagnosis of an organization will be achieved by identifying the business environment it is operating in and the value drivers. This will be performed as follows:

- In-depth interviews with workers and managers

- Examining financial reports, marketing reports, and operational and development reports

- Examining other improvement endeavors (external and internal) of the organization

- Collecting external information on the organization

Once the value drivers have been identified, they are sorted so that we can focus on the more important ones.

Preliminary Implementation Plan

After the business-functional assessment has been completed, a draft is prepared of a value-enhancing implementation plan.

Training and Knowledge Transfer

Knowledge about new management approaches and tools that were described in this book will be transferred to management through an interactive workshop lasting several days. During this workshop, management identifies the value drivers and prepares a detailed implementation plan. At a later date, the knowledge will be transferred to middle management and the rest of the workers.

The guiding principle is that management and the workers themselves will implement the change. This reduces resistance to change because it is done internally and not by external agents.

Value Enhancement Teams

Management should establish value enhancement teams that will deal with the various value drivers. The value-enhancing process is carried out in the spirit and using the tools presented in this book.

Performance, Monitoring, and Control

Management serves as a steering committee for the project. Its role is to oversee and manage the work of the value enhancement teams, meet with them on a regular basis, and approve their findings and recommendations for implementation.

Principles of Introducing Changes and Reducing Resistance to Change

Several principles should guide management when it plans to enhance the value of the organization or improve its performance:

- People within the organization will implement the change.

- The role of an optional external body will be to introduce methods, transfer knowledge to management and workers, and facilitate the implementation process.

- The value enhancement teams will include rank-and-file people of the organization.

- The number of teams will be small, and they will be responsible for suggesting changes and for the actual implementation.

- Areas for enhancement will be chosen by their contribution to value and the difficulty in implementing them, using the focusing matrix.

- Value enhancement plays a central role of the duty and work of management and is not a side project.

- All the organization's workers should gradually join the knowledge transfer circles.

- Follow-up and control of the implementation of value enhancement will be done using the tools presented in this book.

The Role of Information Systems in the Change Process

Information systems play a central role in the change process. However, the idea that implementing an information system will in itself solve an organization's problems is misleading. An information system in an organization should be implemented according to a two-stage model (Ronen and Pass, 1997), as follows:

- *Changing the managerial approaches and the managerial process of the organization:* First, there is a need to implement approaches such as management by constraints; the complete kit concept; the value-focused management model; the three-stage model of decision making, global measuring, and control; project management methods; management of research and development; and more.
- *Designing an information system that will support the above approaches:* After the work processes have been designed and the managerial approaches have been implemented, the information systems must be adapted to support these approaches. The resulting information system designed in a satisficer frame of mind will be highly effective yet simple. Building such information systems to support these approaches is a necessary condition for a continuation of value enhancement processes over time.

Chapter Summary

What will management look like in the future? Management will probably reflect the business, economic, social, technological, and political environments. Management approaches will adapt themselves in the future to changing environments. We believe that as some of the principles presented in this book serve as basic building blocks in the future, new managerial innovations will arise that will illuminate existing and new problems in a way that will provide additional insight about the management world.

References

Borovitz, I., and Ein-Dor, P. "Cost/Utilization: A Measure of System Performance." *Communications of the ACM*, 1977, *20*(3), 185–191.

Burbridge, J. L. *The Principles of Production Control.* (2nd ed.) London: Macdonald & Evans, 1968.

Coman, A., Koller, G., and Ronen, B. "The Application of Focused Management in the Electronics Industry: A Case Study." *Production and Inventory Management*, Second Quarter 1996, pp. 65–70.

Cooper, R., and Kaplan, R. S. "Measure Costs Right: Make the Right Decisions." *Harvard Business Review*, 1988, pp. 96–103.

Copeland, T., Koller, T., and Murrin, J. *Valuation: Measuring and Managing the Value of Companies.* Hoboken, N.J.: Wiley, 1996.

Cox, J. F., III, and Blackstone, J. H. *APICS Dictionary.* (9th ed.) Falls Church, Va.: American Production and Inventory Control Society, 1998.

Cox, J. F., III, and Spencer, M. S. *The Constraint Management Handbook.* Boca Raton, Fla.: St. Lucie Press, 1998.

Crosby, P. B. *Quality Is Free.* New York: McGraw-Hill, 1979.

Czuchry, A. J., Yasin, M. M., and Norris, J. "An Open System Approach to Process Reengineering in a Healthcare Operational Environment." *Health Marketing Quarterly*, 2000, *17*(3), 77–88.

Deming, W. E. *Out of the Crisis.* Cambridge, Mass.: MIT Center for Advanced Engineering Study, 1986.

Dettmer, H. W. *Breaking the Constraints to World-Class Performance.* Milwaukee, Wisc.: American Society for Quality, 1998.

Eden, Y., and Ronen, B. "Improving Workflow in the Insurance Industry: A Focused Management Approach." *Journal of Insurance Issues*, 1993, *16*(1), 49–62.

Eden, Y., and Ronen, B. "Activity-Based Costing and Activity-Based Management." *Articles of Merit 2002 Competition, FMAC Award Programs for Distinguished Contribution of Management Accounting, International Federation of Accounting.* New York: International Federation of Accountants, 2002.

Geri, N., and Ronen, B. "Relevance Lost: The Rise and Fall of Activity-Based Costing." *Human Systems Management,* 2005, *24*(2), 133–144.

Goldratt, E. M. *The Haystack Syndrome: Sifting Information out of the Data Ocean.* Croton-on-Hudson, N.Y.: North River Press, 1990.

Goldratt, E. M. *It's Not Luck.* Croton-on-Hudson, N.Y.: North River Press, 1994.

Goldratt, E. M. *Critical Chain.* Croton-on-Hudson, N.Y.: North River Press, 1997.

Goldratt, E. M., and Cox, J. *The Goal.* (2nd rev. ed.) Croton-on-Hudson, N.Y.: North River Press, 1992.

Goldratt, E. M., and Fox, R. E. *The Race.* Croton-on-Hudson, N.Y.: North River Press, 1986.

Grosfeld-Nir, A., and Ronen, B. "The Complete Kit Concept: Modeling the Managerial Approach." *Computers and Industrial Engineering,* 1998, *34*(3), 695–701.

Hillier, F. S., and Lieberman, G. J. *Introduction to Operations Research.* (7th ed.) New York: McGraw-Hill, 2002.

Hölzer, S., Tafazzoli, A. G., Altmann, U., Wachter, W., and Dudeck, J. "Data Warehousing as a Tool for Quality Management in Oncology." *Studies in Health Technology and Informatics,* 1999, *68,* 432–435.

Horngren, C. T., Foster, G., and Datar, S. M. *Cost Accounting: A Managerial Emphasis.* (10th ed.) Upper Saddle River, N.J.: Prentice Hall, 2000.

Johnson, H. T., and Kaplan, R. S. *Relevance Lost: The Rise and Fall of Management Accounting.* Cambridge, Mass.: Harvard Business School Press, 1987.

Juran, J. M. *Juran on Leadership for Quality.* New York: Free Press, 1989.

Karp, A., and Ronen, B. "Improving Manufacturing Operations: An Entropy Model Approach." *International Journal of Production Research,* 1992, *30*(4), 923–938.

Leshno, M., and Ronen, B. "The Complete Kit Concept—Implementataion in the Health Care System." *Human Systems Management,* 2001, *20*(4), 313–318.

Livne, Z., and Ronen, B. "The Component Chart: A New Tool for Purchasing and Production." *Production and Inventory Management,* First Quarter 1990, pp. 18–23.

Mabin, J. M., and Balderstone, S. J. *The World of the Theory of Constraints: A Review of International Literature.* Boca Raton, Fla.: St. Lucie Press, 2000.

Pass, S., and Ronen, B. "Managing the Market Constraint in the High-Tech Industry." *International Journal of Operations Management*, 2003, *41*(4), 713–724.

Ronen, B. "The Complete Kit." *International Journal of Production Research*, 1992, *30*(10), 2457–2466.

Ronen, B., Coman, A., and Schragenheim, E. "Peak Management." *International Journal of Production Research*, 2001, *39*(14), 3183–3193.

Ronen, B., and Pass, S. "Manufacturing Management Information Systems Require Simplification." *Industrial Engineering*, 1997, *24*(2), 50–53.

Ronen, B., and Spector, Y. "Managing System Constraints: A Cost/Utilization Approach." *International Journal of Production Research*, 1992, *30*(9), 2045–2061.

Ronen, B., and Starr, M. "Synchronized Manufacturing as in OPT: From Practice to Theory." *Computers and Industrial Engineering*, 1990, *18*(8), 585–600.

Schonberger, R. J. *World Class Manufacturing: The Lessons of Simplicity Applied.* New York: Free Press, 1986.

Schragenheim, E., and Ronen, B. "The Drum-Buffer-Rope Shop Floor Control." *Production and Inventory Management*, 1990, *31*(3), 18–23.

Shingo, S. *Quick Changeover for Operators: The SMED System.* Cambridge, Mass.: Productivity Press, 1996.

Simon, H. A. *Models of Man.* Hoboken, N.J.: Wiley, 1957.

Stern, J. M., and Shiely, J. S. *The EVA Challenge.* Hoboken, N.J.: Wiley, 2001.

Stewart, G. B., III. "EVA: Fact and Fantasy." *Journal of Applied Corporate Finance*, 1994, *7*(2), 1078–1196.

Suzaki, K. *The New Manufacturing Challenge.* New York: Free Press, 1987.

Taguchi, G. *Introduction to Quality Engineering: Designing Quality into Products and Processes.* Cambridge, Mass.: Productivity Press, 1986.

Index

A

ABC classification, 30–31
Accounting: activity-based, 245; cost, 237–242, 243t; throughput, 245–246; value driver identification through, 288. *See also* Operating expenses
Acquired infections, 157–159
Activity-based costing, 245
Assessing value, 283–284
Asset value, 284
Automation, 229
Average resource utilization, 144

B

Bad multitasking, 183–185, 184*fig*, 316
Balderstone, S. J., 10, 77
Batches: calculating cost of, 181–182, 241; description of, 172; GMH case study on working with small, 315; JIT Rule II on working with small, 172–182, 234; overview of, 176–182; strategic importance of small, 178–182; transfer, 173–176. *See also* Production
"Bid-no bid" process, 107
Blackstone, J. H., 211
Blood test CUT diagram, 251*fig*–252
Bottlenecks (market constraints): CUT diagram of, 70*fig*; deciding

how to exploit/utilize constraints, 101–108; definition of, 56–57; elevate and break the constraint, 111–112; examples of, 57*fig*–58; exploiting, 102*fig*–106; load analysis in system with, 69t; preventing inertia as becoming, 112–117; steps of management by constraints in case of, 100–117; strategic issues of, 115–116; subordinating system to the constraint, 109–111
Bottlenecks (resource constraints): CUT diagram of, 68*fig*; definition of, 51; discrete events of, 56; distinguishing between noncritical resources and, 239; efficiency/utilization increased to break, 77–80; examples of, 51–52*fig*, 53–54; peak time, 55–56; permanent, 54–55; shortage of critical, 54; strategic issues of, 115–116; work rate of the, 90
Brand name, "stretching" the, 111–112
"Bread-and-butter law," 219–220
Breaking of assumptions (CRD), 136–137
Burbridge, J. L., 187
Business diagnosis, 332
Business environment: adoption of new managerial approaches in,

Business environment, *continued*
8–10; decision making in resource-constrained, 246–248; GDM in excess capacity, 250–261; globalization impact on the, 5–8; management principles in dynamic, 11–27; moving from a sellers' to buyers' market, 4–5; scissors diagram on new pressures of, 7–8*fig*; sellers' market in the, 3–4. *See also* Health care systems; Organizations
Buyers' market: globalization context of, 6–7; moving from sellers' market to, 4–5

C
Capacity: excess, 226, 227, 228, 250–261; nominal, 226; protective, 226–228; traditional approaches to managing fluctuations in, 229; utilization (load analysis) of, 63–65, 66*t*, 68*t*, 69*t*
Car fleet CRD (conflict resolution diagram), 136*fig*
Case studies: Guard Mountain Hospital, 309–322*t*; Queen Medical Center, 292–306*fig*
Cash flow, 155–156
Centrality of the customer, 266, 274
Centralization versus decentralization, 131
CEOs' global decision-making perspective, 86, 249, 251–252, 256, 258
Change: deciding on what and how to, 331; principles of reducing resistance/introducing, 333–334; process of, 331–333; role of information systems in process of, 334
Claims department, 188*fig*
Classification (Pareto focusing method): garbage time causes, 79–80; monitoring drug consumption application, 36–37; purchasing application, 35
Colonoscopy, 198–199
Coman, A., 10, 55, 114, 192

Communication, globalization impact on, 5
Competition (ongoing), 327
Complete kits: definition of, 192; drawbacks of incomplete kit, 192–196; field results of using, 203–204; GMH case study on use of, 316–317; health care system context of, 198–199; implementing in health care organization, 200–202; implications for health management information systems (MIS), 202–203; implications for purchasing and logistics departments, 203; overview of, 191–192; quality management support of, 200; reasons for not using, 196–197; reducing response times/WIP using, 165; theory of constraints support and use of, 200
Computerization, 229
Conflicts. *See* Managerial conflicts
Constraints. *See* System constraints
Continuous improvement in surgical department, 97*fig*
Contract bidding decisions, 248
Control: global performance measures as tool for, 206; improving quality and process, 234; incomplete kit and increased complexity and, 196; orthogonal, 127; to reduce waste, 183; stages in managing quality and process, 268–275. *See also* Quality
Cooper, R., 245
Copeland, T., 287
Core competence matrix, 252–253*fig*
Core problems, 289, 324
Cost accounting: assumptions underlying traditional, 243*t*; dominance of financial accounting over, 239–240; examples of loss of relevance of traditional, 240–242; factors responsible for loss of relevancy, 238–240; loss of relevance of traditional, 237–240; managerial decision making and

activity-based, 245. *See also* CUT (cost-utilization) diagrams; Operating expenses
Cost per unit, 181–182, 241
Cost world, 276–277
Cox, J., 12, 47, 48, 53, 77, 90, 143, 181, 207, 210, 224, 237
Cox, J. F., III, 211, 226
CRD (conflict resolution diagram): breaking assumptions mechanism for, 136–137; on conflict resolution using complete kit, 197*fig*; described, 132; differentiation mechanism used for, 135; drawing a, 133–135, 134*fig*; examples of, 135*fig*, 136*fig*, 137*fig*–141*fig*; globalization of, 135–136; injection used in, 138*fig*–141*fig*. *See also* Managerial conflicts
"Critical chain" approach, 234, 324
Crosby, P. B., 264
CRT (current reality tree). *See f*CRT (focused current reality tree)
Cumulative fluctuations, 224–226*fig*
"Curse of the blessing," 98
Customers: centrality of the, 266, 274; creating added value for the, 112; focus on MVCs (most valuable customers), 112–113; implementing group technology by, 187*fig*; reducing fluctuations by sharing information with, 232; sales effort and specific contribution of, 105*t*; subordinating system to needs of, 109–111; WIP and diminished satisfaction of, 156
CUT (cost-utilization) diagrams: for alternative resource utilization, 222*fig*–233*fig*; for blood tests, 251*fig*–252; defining relative costs of resources in, 65*t*, 67; to depict system and work process, 67*fig*; described, 65; investment decisions using, 71–72; routine use of, 72; of system with market constraint, 70*fig*; of system with resource constraint, 68*fig*–69. *See also* Cost accounting; Operating expenses

D

Datar, S. M., 287
DBR (drum-buffer-rope) mechanism, 90–93, 91*fig*, 183
Decentralization: centralization versus, 131; global performance measures to facilitate, 207
Decision-making: CUT (cost-utilization) diagram used for, 71–72; GDM (global decision-making) method for, 86–87, 249–261; global performance measures to aid, 206; managerial, 245–246; measurements profile tool for global, 216*t*–217; Mirabilis effect and, 85–86; Queen Medical Center case study and value creation, 300–306; in resource-constrained environment, 246–248; satisficers versus optimizers process of, 14–18, 17*fig*
Demand: as function of price, 257*t*; service mix and, 258*fig*
Deming, W. E., 12, 192, 195, 232, 275, 276
Dettmer, H. W., 119
Development-production conflicts, 326
Differentiation (Pareto focusing method): for CRD (conflict resolution diagram), 135; to exploit/utilize policy constraint, 80; managerial frame of mind on, 330–331; monitoring drug consumption application, 37; purchasing application, 35
Discounted cash flow, 284
Discrete events of resource constraints, 56
"Drawer effect," 146–147
Due date performance: using dollar-days measure of, 213*t*; as global performance measure, 212–214; in GMH case study, 311

Dummy constraints: breaking bottlenecks of, 87, 101–108; breaking sales, 107–108; CUT diagram for system with, 71*fig*; definition of, 60; examples of, 60–61; GMH case study on breaking, 316; load analysis for system with, 71*t*

E

Economic approach to quality, 264–266

Economies-of-scale thinking, 181

ED (emergency department): changing organizational structure of the, 303–304; CRDs for, 139*fig*–140*fig*; creating value by improving, 281–282; 40-20-40 phenomenon in, 172; Guard Mountain Hospital case study, 309–322*t*; implementing group technology into, 186, 187–188; incomplete kit and increased WIP in, 193; reducing waiting times in, 302–303; response time in, 152

Eden, Y., 95, 146, 158, 192, 208

Effectiveness: definition of, 76; prioritization and, 82–86; specific contribution to, 83–85*fig*; strategic gating and, 81–83; strategic marketing, 104–106

Efficiencies syndrome: as barrier to using complete kit and, 196–197; causes of, 145–146, 148; dealing with, 147–148; definition of, 143, 144; "drawer effect" of, 146–147; excess WIP due to, 159; illustration of, 143–144

Efficiency: classifying garbage time causes to increase, 79–80; core competence matrix and, 252–253*fig*; definition of, 76; differential policy to increase, 80; increasing constraint utilization and, 77–81; production, 241–242; resource allocation to increase, 80–81

Efficient production, 241–242

85-15 rule, 270, 330

Elevating/breaking system constraints, 93–96

Employees: changing in character of salary costs of, 239; "drawer effect" and, 146–147; efficiencies syndrome and, 143–148, 159, 196–197; 85-15 rule on responsibility of, 270, 330; false "savings" of transferring department, 242; improving human resources for, 304–305; incomplete kit and declining motivation of, 195; incomplete kits as goodwill expression by, 197*fig*; process control participation of, 273–274; WIP and diminished motivation of, 156. *See also* Managers

EVA (economic value-added) measures, 284–287, 286*t*

Evaluation, global performance measures used for, 206

Excess capacity: described, 226, 227, 228; GDM method in environment of, 250–261; how to handle, 257–258, 260–261

Expediting orders, 229

Exploiting constraints: how to utilize and, 87, 101–108; market constraint, 102*fig*–106

External uncertainty, 327

F

fCRT construction: exercising orthogonal control during, 127; identifying core problems of, 126–127; information sources for, 121; principles of, 121; role of undesirable effect in, 126

fCRT (focused current reality tree): advantages and disadvantages of, 127–128; described, 119, 120; example of, 128*fig*; in GMH case study, 317, 318*fig*; inferences of, 126*fig*; objectives of using, 119–

120; Queen Medical Center case study, 299*fig*; routine use of, 128–129; template for, 120*fig*; undesirable effects of, 121–125*fig*; using, 121–127

*f*CRT undesirable effects: as core problem, 126–127; examples of, 124*fig*–125*fig*; importance and logical relations among, 122–124*fig*; list of, 121–122

Final inspections, 230

Finished good inventory, 228, 234

"Fitness to use," 266

Fluctuation evolution: CUT diagrams for resource utilizations, 222*fig*–233*fig*; planned process as part of, 221*fig*; selecting best alternative for organization, 223–226*fig*

Fluctuations: cumulative, 224–226*fig*; described, 219–220; elements of capacity, 226–228; evolution of, 221*fig*–226*fig*; focused management approach to managing, 230–234; internal, 223–224, 225*fig*–226*fig*; protecting against, 231–232; reducing, 232–234; sources of, 220–221; traditional approaches to managing, 228–230

Focused management: classifying problems by contribution to organization, 24*fig*–25; elements of, 18–20; establishing strategy for, 111; of fluctuations in health care system, 230–234; triangle of, 20*fig*–26

Focused management triangle: diagram of, 20*fig*; focusing on essentials, 23–26; global system view, 20–23; simple tools used, 26

Focusing matrix, 38, 39*fig*, 40, 82–83, 306*fig*, 319*t*

Focusing table, 37–38, 39*t*, 82–83, 305*t*, 319*fig*

Ford, H., 88, 96

Ford Motor Company, 96

Forecasting capability, 156–157*fig*

40-20-40 phenomenon, 172

Foster, G., 287

Fox, R. E., 156, 173

G

Garbage plants: examples of, 265; of organization, 327–328; reduction of, 183, 266

Garbage time: classifying causes of, 79–80; definition of, 79; reducing sales force, 102

GDM (global decision-making): adding strategic considerations to, 249–250, 252–254, 256–257, 258; CEO's perspective on, 86, 249, 251–252, 256, 258; description of, 86–87; in excess capacity environment, 250–261; in resource-constrained environment, 246–248; tools used for, 248; types of managerial decisions using, 245–246

Geri, N., 83, 249

Global performance measures: adapted to an OR, 214–216; benefits of, 205–207; described, 205; due date performance as, 212–214; establishing, 49–50; inventory as, 211; measurements profile tool used with, 216*t*–217; operating expenses as, 210–211; quality as, 212; Queen Medical Center case study use of, 297; response time as, 211–212; throughput as, 208–210; types listed, 208; value driver identification through, 289

Global system view: described, 20–21; expanding scope of the system, 21; expanding the time frame, 22–23; managerial frame of mind and, 328

Globalization: buyers' market in context of, 6–7; communication changes influenced by, 5; CRD (conflict resolution diagram), 134*fig*, 135–136; multinational firms resulting from, 5; social and political impact of, 5–6

GMH (Guard Mountain Hospital) case study: adverse effects of WIP in, 313–317; background information on, 309–310; fCRT (focused current reality tree) in, 317, 318fig; focusing matrix used in, 319fig; focusing table used in, 319t; management of system's constraints, 310–313; teams used during, 317, 318fig, 320t–322t

"Go-no go" process, 107

Goldratt, E. M., 12, 47, 48, 53, 77, 90, 119, 132, 143, 156, 173, 181, 207, 210, 224, 237, 245, 276, 331

Grosfeld-Nir, A., 192

Gross response time (throughput time), 153, 157

Group technology, 186fig–189

H

Health care systems: complete kit concept in the, 198–199; focused management approach to fluctuations in, 230–234; need for new managerial approaches to, 3–4; traditional cost accounting loss of relevance for, 240–241. *See also* Business environment; Organizations

Hillier, F. S., 152

Horngren, C. T., 287

Howard Johnson's, 267

Human resources: improving, 304–305; managerial frame of mind and, 329

I

Imaging projects, 84t

In-kit, 192

Inherent conflicts, 326

Injection (CRD): described, 137; examples of, 138fig–141fig

Input-output model, 9fig–10

Inspection, 269fig

Internal fluctuations, 223–224, 225fig–226fig

Internal uncertainty, 327

Inventories: excess WIP due to perceived assets of, 159; finished goods, 228, 234; as global performance measurement, 211; raw material, 150fig, 230, 234; types of, 149–150fig. *See also* WIPs (works in process)

Investment decisions, 247

J

JIT Rule I: applied to shortage deviation, 167; applied to surplus deviation, 168–169; definition of, 166–167; 40-20-40 phenomenon created by, 172; implementing for maintenance, 169; implementing in scheduling tasks/meetings, 169–170; violations of, 170fig–172

JIT Rule II: applied to transfer batches, 173–176; applied to working (production) batches, 176–179; definition of, 172; determination of batch size for, 173; for reducing response times/working with small batches, 179–182, 234

JIT Rule III: to avoid wastes, 182–183; methods used to eliminate waste under, 183–189

Johnson, H. T., 237

Juran, J. M., 266

K

Kaplan, R. S., 237, 245

Karp, A., 181

Killer, T., 287

Knowledge gap, 159

Knowledge transfer, 332

Koller, G., 10, 192

L

LCC (life-cycle cost), 136

Leshno, M., 192

Level of aspiration, 16–17

Lieberman, G. J., 152

"Life-cycle cost," 22

"Line balancing" concept, 228
Livne, Z., 36
Load analysis (capacity utilization): effect of batch size on load of non-critical resources, 180t; examples of, 66t, 68t, 69t; management during peak-time loads, 113–115; overview of, 63–65
Local optimization, 14
Logistics department, 203

M

Mabin, J. M., 10, 77
McDonald's, 264, 267
Make-or-buy decisions, 247, 252t
Management: adoption of new managerial approaches by, 8–10; challenge of creating value, 281–282; complete kit concept and quality, 200; 85-15 rule on responsibility of, 270, 330; focused, 18–26, 230–234; process control commitment of, 274; satisficer versus optimizer approach to, 14–18; scissors diagram of pressures on, 7–8fig; stages in quality and process control, 268–275; traditional approach to fluctuations, 228–230; VFM (value-focused management) model of, 287–290
Management by constraints: seven-step process of, 47–48, 100; step 1: determine the system's goal, 48–49; step 2: establish global performance measures, 49–50; step 3: identify the system constraint, 50–72; step 4: decide how to exploit/utilize the constraint, 75–87, 101–108; step 5: subordinate the system to the constraint, 87–93, 109–111; step 6: elevate and break the constraint, 93–96, 111–112; step 7: if constraint is "broken" go back to step 3, 96–98, 112–117
Managerial conflicts: definition of, 131, 132; development-production,

326; examples of, 131, 135fig–141fig; inherent, 326; routine use of conflict resolution approach to, 142; steps in dealing with, 133fig–141fig. See also CRD (conflict resolution diagram)
Managerial credo: implementing focused management methods, 331; managerial frame of mind and, 323–330; principles of introducing changes/reducing resistance to change, 333–334; on process of change, 331–333; role of information systems in change process, 334
Managerial frame of mind: all organizations are "sick," 325–328; differentiation and, 330–331; 85-15 rule and, 270, 330; human resources and, 329; managerial maturity, 328–329; using performance measures, 330; satisficer principle and, 329–330; using simple tools, 330; taking a global view, 328; ten times rule and, 272–273fig, 330; "the world is simpler than it seems," 323–325
Managerial maturity, 328–329
Managers: decision-making processes taken by, 245–262; process control participation of, 273–274; value creation from activities of, 282–283; WIP and diminished motivation of, 156. See also Employees
Market: product differentiation and segmentation of, 110–111, 248, 260–261; role of demand in, 257t, 258fig; subordinating technology to needs of, 110; TTM (time to market) of services and products, 103; WIP and diminished flexibility to changes in, 155
Market constraints: CUT diagram of, 70fig; definition of, 56–57; examples of, 57fig–58; exploiting, 102fig–106; load analysis in system

Market constraints, *continued* with, 69t; steps of management by constraints in case of, 100–117; strategic issue of, 115–116

Market value, 283

Marketing: effectiveness of strategic, 104–106; segmentation, 110–111, 248

Measurements profile: for make-or-buy decision, 252t; overview of, 216t–217; for production example, 256t; of service mix example, 259t. *See also* Performance measurements

Meeting scheduling, 169–170

Mirabilis effect, 85–86

MIS (management information system): complete kit implications for, 202–203; role in change process, 334

Model T Ford, 88

Multinational firms, 5

Multitasking (bad), 183–185, 184fig, 316

Murphy's Law, 219–220

Murrin, J., 287

Mushroom effect, 233fig–234

MVCs (most valuable customers), 112–113

N

New managerial approaches: characteristics of, 9; input-output model of, 9fig–10; pressures leading to adoption of, 3–9

Nominal capacity, 226

NOPAT (net operating profit after taxes), 284–286

O

Offloading: described, 94–95; examples of, 95–96; in GMH case study, 313

Ongoing competition, 327

Operating expenses: calculating profit using, 214; cost per unit, 181–182, 241; global performance measure-ment of, 210–211; LCC (life-cycle cost), 136; long response time and high operating, 154; NOPAT (net operating profit after taxes), 284–286; reduction of, 103–104; selecting best alternative for resource costs, 223–226fig; value created from discounted cash flow, 284. *See also* Accounting; Cost accounting; CUT (cost-utilization) diagrams

Operational approach to quality, 264

Optimization, 13

Optimizers: decision-making of satisfi-cers versus, 17fig–18; definition of, 15; management approach taken by, 15–16

OR (operating room): CRDs (conflict resolution diagrams) for, 139fig, 141fig; creating value by improving, 281; global performance measures adapted to, 214–216; implementing group technology into, 186fig–187fig; incomplete kit and increased response time in, 193–194; increasing throughput of, 300–301

Organizations: business diagnosis of, 332; classifying problems by contri-bution to, 24fig–25; conflict between goals of individuals and, 326–327; core competence matrix of, 252–253fig; "curse of the bless-ing" and, 98; effect of reducing WIP on, 161fig; implementing complete kit in health care, 200–202; managerial frame of mind on "sick," 325–328. *See also* Busi-ness environment; Health care sys-tems; Systems; Value

Orthogonal control, 127

O'Toole principle, 220

Out-kit, 192

Outpatient clinic throughput, 304

Overproduction (spares), 229

P

Pareto diagram: building, 34; drug use in a hospital example of, 31–34; prioritization using, 82, 85*fig*; of specific contribution, 85*fig*; steps for deriving, 31

Pareto focusing matrix, 38, 39*fig*, 40, 82–83, 306*fig*, 319*t*

Pareto focusing table, 37–38, 39*t*, 82–83, 305*t*, 319*fig*

Pareto rule: ABC classification expansion of the, 30–31; described, 29; focusing method application of, 34–37; focusing table and focusing matrix applications of, 37–40; management phenomena following the, 29–30; recommendations for using, 42–43; solutions to implementation failures of, 42; use, misuse, and abuse of the, 40–42

Pareto, V., 29

Pareto-based focusing method: monitoring drug consumption application of, 36–37; overview of, 34–35; purchasing application of, 35–36

Pass, S., 55, 100, 165, 334

Peak-time loads: management during, 113–115, 316; resource constraints during, 55–56

Performance measurements: due date, 212–214, 213*t*; EVA (economic value-added), 284–287, 286*t*; GDM method and changes in local, 249–250, 255, 257, 261; global decision-making and measuring local, 87; global performance, 49–50, 205–216, 289, 297; managerial frame of mind and use of, 330; Queen Medical Center case study, 293; VFM model and determining, 288

Policies: conflict between opposing, 131; relationship between performance measures and, 205–206

Policy constraints (or policy failure): breaking bottlenecks of, 87,

101–108; breaking sales, 107–108; control test of, 60; definition of, 58; examples of, 58–60; in GMH case study, 312

Prices: decisions on, 247–248; demand as function of, 257*t*. *See also* Purchasing

Prioritization methods: in bid-no bid processes, 107; using focusing table and focusing matrix, 82–83; Mirabilis effect, 85–86; using Pareto diagram, 82, 85*fig*; using specific contribution, 83–85*fig*

Problems: classifying by contribution to organization, 24*fig*–25; core, 289, 324; 85-15 rule on responsibility for, 270, 330; fluctuations resulting in, 219–235; orthogonal control to identify, 127; process control approach to solving, 271–275; product mix, 246–247; ten-times rule on, 272–273*fig*; UDEs (undesirable effects) of *f*CRT as, 121–127

Process flow diagram, 62–63*fig*, 64*fig*

Product mix problem, 246–247

Production: efficiency, 241–242; GDM method for decisions regarding, 255–257; handling excess of capacity in, 257–258, 260–261; measurements profiles for, 256*t*. *See also* Batches

Products: avoiding sale of "complete or nothing," 108; conflict between limited versus large variety of, 131; "critical chain" approach to, 234; decisions to introduce new, 247; expanding variety of, 239; final inspection and sorting of, 230; generic versus custom, 131; implementing group technology by, 187*fig*; improving quality of, 103; market segmentation and differentiation of, 110–111, 248, 260–261; mushroom effect for, 233*fig*–234; overproduction (spares), 229; repairs to, 230; separate line for

Products, *continued*
every, 233*fig*; TTM (time to market) of, 103. *See also* Quality;
Response times; Services; WIPs
(works in process)
Profit calculation, 214
Protective capacity, 226–228
Purchasing: classification (Pareto
focusing method) applied to, 35;
differentiation (Pareto focusing
method) applied to, 35; dummy
constraints due to decisions in,
60–61; implications of complete kit
concept for, 203; policy constraints
applied to, 58–60; reducing costs of,
304. *See also* Prices

Q

Quality: centrality of the customer
and, 266, 274; controlling waste by
improving, 183; definitions of,
263–268; economic approach to,
264–266; as global performance
measure, 212; in GMH case study,
311; implementing processes for
improving, 275–276; improving
service and product, 103; incomplete kit resulting in poor, 194; long
response time and diminished,
154–155; myths about improving,
277; operational approach to, 264;
stages in managing process control
and, 268–275; strategic leverage of
excellence in, 106–107; traditional
approaches to managing fluctuations in, 229–230; uniformity
approach to, 266–268. *See also*
Control; Products; Services
Quality improvement myths, 277
Quality management: complete kit
concept and, 200; implementing
improvement processes, 275–276;
stage one: organization has no quality management/feedback, 268;
stage three: process control,

269–275; stage two: inspection of
quality control, 269*fig*; throughput
world and cost world objectives of,
276–277
Queen Medical Center case study:
background information on,
292–293; focused current reality
tree for, 299*fig*; focusing matrix for
value enhancement in, 306*fig*;
focusing table for value drivers in,
305*t*; improvement implementing
process, 305–306; step 1: determining value creation goal, 293; step 2:
determining performance measures,
293; step 3: identification of value
drivers, 293–298, 300; step 4: deciding how to improve value drivers,
300–305; SWOT analysis of, 295*t*

R

Rate of market demand, 90
Raw materials: definition of, 150*fig*;
standardizing components and,
234; traditional management of
fluctuations in, 230
Repairs, 230
Resource allocation (Pareto focusing
method): exploit/utilize resource
constraint, 80; monitoring drug
consumption application, 37; purchasing application, 36
Resource constraints (or bottleneck):
CUT diagram of, 68*fig*; decision
making in environment of,
246–248; definition of, 51; discrete
events of, 56; effect of batch size on
load of noncritical, 180*t*; effi-
ciency/utilization increased to
break, 77–80; examples of,
51–52*fig*, 53–54; peak time, 55–56;
permanent, 54–55; shortage of critical, 54; strategic issues of, 115–117
Resource utilization: considering elements of capacity, 226–228; CUT
diagrams for alternative,

222fig–223fig; protecting against fluctuations in, 230–234; selecting best alternative for, 223–226fig; traditional approaches to managing fluctuations and, 228–230

Resources: distinguishing between bottlenecks and noncritical, 239; elements of capacity, 226–228; fluctuations and utilization of, 223–234; focused managed approach to fluctuations and, 230–234; traditional approaches to making fluctuations and, 228–230

Response time reduction: JIT Rule I, 166–172; JIT Rule II for, 172–182; JIT Rule III for, 182–183; management by constraints for, 166; methods listed, 164; strategic gating for, 164–165; strategic importance of, 179–182; working with complete kit, 165

Response times: as barrier to using complete kit, 197; as global performance measure, 211–212; in GMH case study, 311; improved in relation to market needs, 103–104; incomplete kit and increase of, 193–194; of 1-2-3 system with transfer batch of 5 units, 175Fig; of 1-2-3 system with transfer batch of 25 units, 174fig; reducing, 163–189; reducing fluctuations by reducing, 232; relation between WIP level and, 152–159; strategic leverage of excellence in, 106–107; UDEs (undesirable effects) of long, 153–159. See also Products; Services

Rewards: global performance measures used for, 206; recommendations for sales personnel, 108

ROA (return on assets), 286t

Ronen, B., 10, 36, 47, 55, 83, 95, 100, 114, 158, 165, 181, 192, 208, 246, 249, 334

S

Salary costs, 239

Sales: breaking policy and dummy constraints to, 107–108; special, 228–229; specific contribution of customers to, 105t

Sales personnel: exploiting marketing and, 102fig–103; recommendations for rewarding, 108; reducing garbage time of, 102

Satisficer principle, 329–330

Satisficers: decision-making of optimizer versus, 17fig–18; definition of, 16; management approach taken by, 16fig–17

Schonberger, R. J., 191, 193, 264

Schragenheim, E., 55, 114

Scissors diagram, 7–8fig

Seasonality resource constraints, 56

Sellers' market: business responses to, 3–4; moving to buyers' market from, 4–5

Services: conflict between limited versus large variety of, 131; decision on stopping production or ceasing, 247; decisions to introduce new, 247; expanding variety of, 239; GDM method for decisions regarding, 255–257; handling excess of capacity in, 257–258, 260–261; improving quality of, 103; measurements profile for example of, 259t; TTM (time to market) of, 103. See also Products; Quality; Response times; WIPs (works in process)

Shareholders' value. See Value

Shiely, J. S., 286

Shingo, S., 180

"Sick" organizations, 325–328

Simon, H. A., 14, 16, 329

Software development CRD (conflict resolution diagram), 137Fig

Special sales, 228–229

Specific contributions: calculating, 83; of customers relative to sales

Specific contributions, *continued*
effort, 105*t*; definition of, 83–84;
examples of, 84–85; Pareto diagram
of, 85*fig*
Spencer, M. S., 212, 226
Staff. *See* Employees
Starr, M., 47
Stern, J. M., 286
Stewart, G. B., III, 285
Strategic considerations (GDM
method), 249, 252–254, 256–257,
258
Strategic gating: calculating specific
contribution to, 83–85; definition
of, 81; examples of, 81–82; in
GMH case study, 314; mirabilis
effect and, 85–86; prioritization
methods for, 82–83; reducing
response times/WIP by, 164–165
Strategic value drivers, 290–292
Suboptimization, 14
Subordination mechanisms: drum-
buffer-rope mechanism, 90–93, 91*fig*;
tactical gating mechanism, 89–90
"Sunk-cost" effect, 59
Suppliers: process control by working
with small number of, 274–275;
reducing fluctuations by sharing
information with, 232
Surgical department continuous
improvement, 97*fig*
Suzaki, K., 191
System constraint tools: Complete
kits, 165, 191–204; CUT (cost-utilization) diagram, 65–72; *f*CRT
(focused current reality tree),
119–129; load analysis, 63–65, 66*t*,
68*t*, 69*t*; overview of, 61–62;
process flow diagram, 62–63*fig*,
64*fig*; time analysis, 63, 64*fig*
System constraints: definition of, 13,
50; elevate and break the, 93–96,
111–112; exploiting/utilizing,
75–87, 101–108, 313; GMH
(Guard Mountain Hospital) management of, 310–313; identifying

the, 50–61; location of, 115–117;
subordinating the system to the,
87–93, 109–111; theory of constraints support on, 200; tools used
to identify, 61–72. *See also specific
constraints*
Systems: change process and role of
information, 334; description of,
11–13; determining goal of, 48–49;
effects of fluctuations, variability,
and uncertainty on, 219–235;
global system view, 20–23, 328;
optimization and suboptimization
of, 13–14; subordinated to the constraint, 87–93; traditional organizational, 12*fig*. *See also* Organizations

T
Tactical gating: described, 89–90; in
GMH case study, 314–316; reducing response time/WIP by, 165
Taguchi, G., 266
Tasks: avoiding bad multitasking to
complete, 183–185, 184*fig*, 316;
DBR (drum-buffer-rope) mechanism to schedule, 90–93, 91*fig*, 183;
finished goods or completed, 150*fig*,
228; in-kit and out-kit of, 192; JIT
Rule I to schedule, 169–170; knowingly forgoing, 328–329; raw material or preprocessing, 150*fig*, 230.
See also WIPs (works in process)
Teams: action items for, 320*t*–322*t*;
creation of, 317; detailed mission
for each, 318*fig*; value enhancement, 333
Technological innovation, 327
Technology: automation and full
computerization, 229; as core competence of organization,
252–253*fig*; implementing group,
186*fig*–189; Queen Medical Center
use of, 296; WIP and diminished
flexibility to changes in, 155
Ten-plus-ten approach, 93
Ten-times rule, 272–273*fig*, 330

Theory of constraints support, 200

Throughput: calculating profit using, 214; calculation of, 209t; definition of, 208; excess WIP and diminished, 157; as global performance measure, 208–210; in GMH case study, 310; incomplete kit and decline in, 195; increasing OR, 300–301; increasing outpatient clinic, 304

Throughput accounting, 245–246

Throughput time (gross response time), 153

Throughput world, 276–277

Time analysis, 63, 64fig

Traffic light zones, 315fig–316

Training transfer, 332

Transaction value, 283–284

Transfer batches, 173–176

TTM (time to market), 103

20-80 rule: ABC classification expansion of, 30–31; applications of, 29–30

Two-dimensional process flow diagram, 64fig

Type A problems, 24fig, 25, 324

Type B problems, 24fig

Type C problems, 24fig, 25

Type D problems, 24fig, 25

U

UDEs (undesirable effects): of fCRT, 121–127; of long response time, 153–159; of utilization), 144–145

UDEs (undesirable effects of fCRT): as core problem, 126–127; examples of, 124fig–125fig; importance and logical relations among, 122–124fig; list of, 121–122

Uncertainty: fluctuations related to, 219–228; focused management approach to managing, 230–234; organizational external and internal, 327; traditional approaches to managing fluctuations and, 228–230

Uniformity approach, 266–268

Utilization: average resource, 144; breaking policy/dummy constraints to increase, 87, 101–108; classifying garbage time causes to increase, 79–80; differential policy to increase, 80; fluctuations and resource, 223–234; increasing constraint, 77–80; resource allocation to increase, 80; resource capacity and, 226–228; undesirable effects of, 144–145

V

Value: assessing firm, 283–284; business goal of increasing shareholder, 48; created from managerial activities, 282–283; effect of reducing WIP on organization, 161fig; EVA (economic value-added) measures of, 284–287, 286t; management challenge of creating, 281–282; Queen Medical Center case study on adding, 292–306fig; VFM (value-focused management) model for increasing, 287–290. See also Organizations

Value drivers: definition of, 19, 288; examples of, 19–20; Queen Medical Center case study, 293–298, 300; strategic, 290–292; top-down approach to, 297–298; VFM model and identification of, 288–290

Value enhancement: definition of, 9; teams for, 333

Value inhibitors, 331

VFM (value-focused management) model: Queen Medical Center case study of, 292–306fig; steps in, 287–290; two dimensions of, 287

W

Wastes: JIT Rule III on avoiding, 182–183; methods used to eliminate, 183–189; types of, 182

WIP reduction: in GMH case study, 314; JIT Rule I for, 166–172; JIT

WIP reduction, *continued*
Rule II for, 172–182; JIT Rule III
for, 182–183; management by constraints for, 166; methods listed,
164; strategic gating for, 164–165
WIPs (works in process): adverse
effects in GMH case study,
310–317; causes of excess, 159; definition of, 150; examples of,
150–151; as global performance
measurement, 211; high-WIP center versus low-WIP center,
151*fig*–162; incomplete kit and
increase of, 193; methods for reducing, 163–189; organizational effect
of reducing, 161*fig*; relation
between response time and level of,
152–159; traditional approaches to
managing fluctuations in, 229;
working with small batches to
improve, 172–182, 234. *See also*
Inventories; Products; Services;
Tasks
Work rate of the bottleneck, 90
Working with complete kit. *See* Complete kits
Working (production) batches. *See*
Batches